Bottom Line's The Healing Kitchen LIBRARY

Popular "Health Foods" That Make You SICK

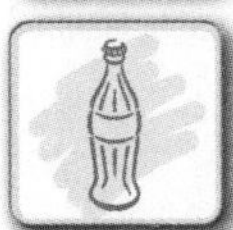

Food Lies & Dirty Labeling Tricks

Best-Ever Healing Herbs & Spices

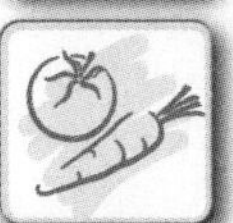

Best-Ever Healing Food Combinations

The Truth About Vitamins & Supplements: The Lifesavers & the Money Wasters

Cooking Secrets That Boost Nutrition

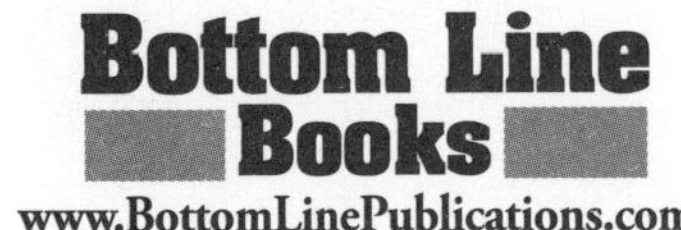
Bottom Line Books
www.BottomLinePublications.com

Bottom Line's The Healing Kitchen Library

First printing

Bottom Line Books® publishes the advice of expert authorities in many fields. These opinions may at times conflict as there are often different approaches to solving problems. The use of this material is no substitute for health, legal, accounting or other professional services. Consult competent professionals for answers to your specific questions.

Telephone numbers, addresses, prices, offers and Web sites listed in this book are accurate at the time of publication, but they are subject to frequent change.

Bottom Line Books® is a registered trademark of
Boardroom® Inc.
281 Tresser Boulevard, Stamford, CT 06901

www.bottomlinepublications.com

Bottom Line Books® is an imprint of Boardroom® Inc., publisher of print periodicals, e-letters and books. We are dedicated to bringing you the best information from the most knowledgeable sources in the world. Our goal is to help you gain greater wealth, better health, more wisdom, extra time and increased happiness.

Printed in the United States of America

HK/am

Contents

SPECIAL REPORT #5:

THE TRUTH ABOUT VITAMINS & SUPPLEMENTS: THE LIFESAVERS & THE MONEY WASTERS

SPECIAL REPORT #6:

COOKING SECRETS THAT BOOST NUTRITION

SPECIAL REPORT #1

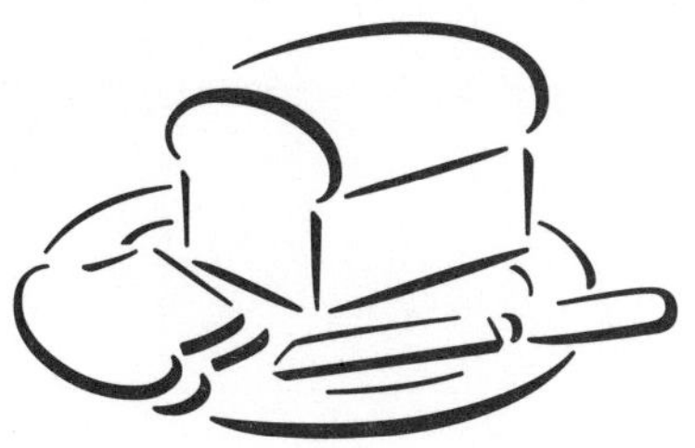

Popular "Health Foods" That Make You Sick

Popular "Health Foods" That Make You Sick

The Inside Scoop on Recent E. Coli Outbreak—How to Protect Yourself

In spring 2011, a particularly virulent type of E. coli—the popular name for *Escherichia coli*—descended upon Europe, primarily hitting Germany, but also striking residents around the continent who had made recent visits to that country. Fifty people from 15 countries succumbed to the disease, which is a record for known E. coli epidemics. The scary thing about this strain is that it acted in a way unlike traditional E. coli and it did not respond to standard treatments.

SUPER TOXIC AND PREVIOUSLY UNKNOWN

This previously unknown variant of E. coli, which scientists describe as a "super toxic" mutant, can cause severe, bloody diarrhea and *hemolytic uremic syndrome* (HUS), a potentially fatal kidney ailment. Beyond the individuals who have died, more than 4,000 people have been sickened, and around 25% developed the dangerous kidney complication—compared with the usual 2% to 7% with other types of E. coli. In another unusual twist, many of the people who became ill were not old and vulnerable, but young adults in the prime of their lives, and the majority were women.

Scientists first suspected Spanish-grown cucumbers, tomatoes and leafy greens, and then bean sprouts from a single organic farm in northern Germany as the culprit. Researchers eventually determined that the contamination began in Egypt, where either human or animal feces came into contact with fenugreek seeds. People became sick from eating fenugreek sprouts.

While there's no need to stop eating fresh fruits and vegetables in the US—we import very little fresh produce from Europe—this outbreak is definitely a wake-up call, warns Andrew L. Rubman, ND, founder and director

Andrew L. Rubman, ND, founder and director, Southbury Clinic for Traditional Medicines, Southbury, Connecticut. *www.southburyclinic.com.*

of Southbury Clinic for Traditional Medicines in Southbury, Connecticut. "E. coli outbreaks and other foodborne illnesses happen all the time—some more virulent than others. As frightening as the headlines are, there are things you can do to protect yourself," he says. Unfortunately, mainstream medicine does not generally have tools to treat this disease beyond managing the symptoms. "This is where naturopathic medicine shines," Dr. Rubman says, "since it helps the body to maximize its own defense mechanisms to fight off illness the way that it is meant to do." Here Dr. Rubman describes what we can do to prevent foodborne disease and how to cope with suspicious symptoms.

DEALING WITH E. COLI THE NATUROPATHIC WAY

If you experience fever, diarrhea and vomiting (the classic signs of E. coli), see your doctor promptly. If there are traces of blood in your stool or vomit, go to the ER.

Meanwhile, since none of us is bullet-proof, here are ways to keep your immune and digestive systems in optimal health and to give yourself a better chance to prevent foodborne illness from striking in the first place...

• **Avoid drugs that make you vulnerable.** If you're a poor eater or a frequent antibiotic user, you weaken your immune defenses and put yourself at greater risk for foodborne and other infections. Frequent use of antibiotics kills off healthful flora in the gut along with the bad, opening the door for nasty organisms like E. coli to overtake your body. Similarly, Dr. Rubman strongly advises against regular use of antacids. One key job of stomach acid is to kill the germs that exist on everything that enters your mouth. Without sufficient stomach acid to kill them, germs are able to infiltrate your system.

• **Pop a probiotic.** Probiotics promote a positive gut ecosystem, allowing the "good bacteria" to flourish so that your body is better able to fend off attacks from incoming toxins.

Dr. Rubman often prescribes: Omega Probiotic from Nordic Naturals (*www.nordicnaturals.com*), which combines probiotics with the omega-3 essential fatty acids EPA and DHA to promote gastrointestinal health and discourage inflammation.

• **Add healthful protein.** Whey protein, derived from cow's milk, can help build up your body's supply of *mucin*, a protective substance in mucus that prevents noxious bacteria from attaching to the lining of the large intestine.

Dr. Rubman often prescribes: Any inexpensive package of whey protein. Purchase it in any health-food store, stir into water and drink, following the package directions. For extra punch, add one teaspoon (about four grams) of vitamin C. Your physician may prescribe larger and more frequent doses of whey protein if you are ill. For those who can't tolerate cow's milk protein, consider goat's milk whey protein isolate.

IF YOU DO GET SICK

When prevention fails and you become ill, naturopathic medicine continues to offer help...

• **Consider botanicals.** Herbs such as echinacea and myrrh have been used for thousands of years to ward off disease.

Dr. Rubman often prescribes: Vita Biotic from Eclectic Institute (*www.eclecticherb.com*), which combines vitamins A and C, echinacea, ginger, garlic, myrrh and more to help strengthen local immunity against insult.

• **Take Western Larch.** Powder from the bark of Western Larch trees, which grow in the Pacific Northwest, enhances immune function in the gut and makes it less vulnerable to microbes.

Dr. Rubman often prescribes: Larix from Eclectic Institute (*www.eclecticherb.com*). Mix one teaspoon to one tablespoon with two to eight ounces of water or unsweetened juice, stir and drink.

• **Other things you can do.** If you develop diarrhea or other digestive upset, it's critical to stay hydrated and to replenish salt and albumin.

Dr. Rubman recommends: Counter dehydration with electrolyte water (such as Pedialyte) and—Dr. Rubman's personal favorite—egg drop soup, which in addition to water is also packed with salt and albumin (the three things that are lost in greatest concentration when you have diarrhea).

Dr. Rubman emphasizes that there is no 100% effective way to guarantee food safety, and the threat of foodborne illnesses will always be with us. Bacteria continuously mutate and adapt to antibiotics, giving rise to nasty new antibiotic-resistant "superbugs" like the one that struck Europe. To protect yourself, be aware, wash your hands frequently, practice safe food handling (e.g., always wash fresh produce thoroughly) and—most important—maintain your own optimal health to counter these ongoing threats.

How to Avoid Unsafe Foods

Rebecca Shannonhouse, editor, *Bottom Line/Health* newsletter, 281 Tresser Boulevard, Stamford, Connecticut 06901.

What do beef, poultry, eggs, spices, fresh spinach and iceberg lettuce all have in common? The FDA allows these foods to be irradiated—that is X-rays or other types of radiation are used to kill harmful organisms that may cause food poisoning.

Immediate danger: In the US, up to 76 million Americans experience some degree of food poisoning each year—and about 5,000 die as a result.

Even so, irradiation has not entirely caught on in the US. It is used only in limited instances—largely because food manufacturers worry about a backlash from consumers.

Some food advocacy groups warn that long-term use of the technology may harm humans, citing research suggesting that animals that have eaten irradiated diets suffered brain damage and other problems as a result.

But the World Health Organization has concluded that irradiation presents no health risks to humans. At the levels that are approved for use in foods, irradiation does not accumulate toxins in the food or generally change the taste of the food, explains Bradley P. Marks, PhD, a food-science and engineering researcher at Michigan State University.

By law, only packaged foods can be irradiated, and they must carry the "radura" symbol (see image at right) on the package. If you prefer to avoid irradiated foods, do not buy items with the radura symbol or...opt for foods that have been labeled "organic"—they have not been irradiated.

Buy at farmers' markets—where you're unlikely to find irradiated foods.

Beware of These Packaged Foods And Drinks

Olga Naidenko, PhD, a senior scientist with the Washington, DC–based Environmental Working Group, *www.ewg.org*, a nonprofit, research-based organization dedicated to protecting public health and the environment. She specializes in the effects of toxic chemicals on human health.

When you buy a food product, you probably don't give much thought to the lining of the food cans, for example, or other material used for packaging. But you should be aware that some materials used to package popular food and beverages are potentially dangerous. *For example...*

- **Candy bars, fast food, microwave popcorn, stick butter and take-out pizza.** These fatty foods are frequently packaged in materials made with a grease-resistant coating that contains *perfluorooctanoic acid* (PFOA), a chemical commonly used in stain-and water-resistant coatings.

Problem: Traces of PFOA invariably remain from the manufacturing process, according to an FDA study. PFOA is highly toxic, and once ingested, it remains in your body for years.

Animal studies have linked it to increased risk for liver, pancreatic and testicular cancers, birth defects and developmental problems, a weakened immune system and elevated total cholesterol.

Self-defense: Avoid any foods wrapped in grease-resistant paper.

Ask restaurant personnel to put food directly in a paper bag (or to wrap it in foil first, for some foods) without the usual grease-resistant paper wrap or cardboard containers (especially when ordering egg breakfast sandwiches, French fries and chicken nuggets—all of which tested highest in PFOA levels in one study). Never heat foods in grease-resistant paper—this increases PFOA exposure.

When heating food in the microwave, I prefer covering it with waxed paper instead of plastic wrap (if it's natural waxed paper and not chemically treated grease-resistant paper wrap). Use foil only when not heating food in a microwave.

Also avoid microwave-ready popcorn—the bags have PFOA in the lining. Instead, buy loose popcorn and pop it on the stovetop in a pot with a small amount of oil or use an electric hot-air popper. If you can't avoid packaging that's grease-resistant, as with store-bought butter, take it out of the wrapping immediately and store in a glass or ceramic container.

• **Bottled beverages and canned foods and beverages.** *Bisphenol A* (BPA) is a component of hard, clear polycarbonate plastics that are used for bottled water and beverages and in the linings of many canned foods.

While BPA, unlike PFOA, is excreted from the body, 93% of Americans who have been tested have traces of BPA in their urine, according to a recent government analysis.

BPA's health risks stem from its estrogen-like effects while in the body. Animal studies have linked BPA exposure to reproductive problems, including miscarriage, infertility and birth defects, as well as increased risk for breast and prostate cancers, liver damage, cardiovascular disease, diabetes and metabolic and nerve disorders.

BPA is present in many beverage bottles and five-gallon water-cooler bottles, as well as the epoxy lining of many food and beverage cans. Canned chicken soup and ravioli are the worst offenders.

Also dangerous: Canned tomatoes. That's because tomatoes' high acid content causes BPA to leach into the food more readily, as well as the cans of any kind of food that have been on the shelf for a long time. While no such period has been defined, scientists know that the leaching of BPA from can linings is an ongoing process while cans are in supermarkets or stored at home.

Self-defense: Limit your consumption of canned foods and beverages, substituting fresh produce or products in glass containers whenever possible. Eden Organic (888-424-3336, *www.edenfoods.com*) is one company now using BPA-free lining for most of its canned foods. Tomatoes are available in protective white enamel-lined cans with minute levels of BPA.

Finally, avoid drinking from plastic beverage bottles or five-gallon plastic water-cooler bottles with the numeral "7" in the recycling triangle on the bottom of the bottle or the letters "PC" (for polycarbonate).

For those concerned about tap-water quality, the best option is to install a water filter. (Learn about filtration systems at *www.ewg.org/tap-water/*).

• **Food and drinks packaged in Styrofoam.** *Polystyrene* (found in Styrofoam food and beverage containers) has been found to leach into liquids and food—particularly in the presence of heat, fats, acid or alcohol. Polystyrene invariably contains residual traces of the chemical *styrene*, which has been linked to nerve damage and cancer risk.

Self-defense: Don't drink beverages from Styrofoam cups—especially heated liquids such as coffee, tea (particularly tea with lemon, which appears to increase leaching) or hot chocolate…fatty liquids, such as milk…or alcoholic drinks.

The same goes for fatty liquids, such as olive oil or oil-based sauces and dressings, which also should not be stored in Styrofoam.

Avoid meats and other foods packaged with Styrofoam backing. When ordering take-out food, request non-Styrofoam containers. Never microwave food in Styrofoam.

Important: It may seem difficult to follow all of this advice all of the time, but you are likely to benefit from just being aware of the risks and limiting your exposure whenever possible.

The BPA Threat—How To Keep This Toxic Chemical Out Of Your Food

Frederick S. vom Saal, PhD, the curators' professor of biological sciences at the University of Missouri in Columbia. He is a leading researcher on the effects of BPA and has conducted dozens of studies on this topic.

Were you relieved by the FDA's recent about-face on bisphenol-A (BPA), the toxic chemical that can leach out of plastic containers and into food? At last, the agency has expressed "some concern" regarding the dangers of this ubiquitous contaminant.

With luck, the FDA's new interest in BPA is not too little too late—but you can also take steps to protect yourself.

BPA is used in many plastic food and beverage containers, particularly those made of hard, clear polycarbonate plastic. BPA is also an additive in *polyvinyl chloride* (PVC) plastic, which is used in some plastic food wraps.

Surprising news: BPA is in the epoxy resins found in the lining of almost all cans used by the food industry (including baby formula cans!). In fact, canned food is the primary food source of BPA for adults.

The problem: BPA molecules that escape their chemical bonds can migrate into the foods and beverages they contact, especially if the container is heated or the food inside is acidic. We then ingest the BPA—thereby increasing our risk for numerous health problems. There's even BPA on the coated paper from cash registers—the toxin gets into our bodies when we touch the paper and then handle the food we're about to eat. BPA can also be absorbed through the skin.

Frederick S. vom Saal, PhD, curators' professor of biological sciences at the University of Missouri and a leading BPA researcher, explained that this chemical has estrogen-like effects on the body. It acts as an endocrine disruptor, interrupting our hormonal patterns—and actually reprogramming our genes. Roughly 1,000 published, peer-reviewed studies have linked BPA to negative health consequences. *These include...*

- **Breast cancer, ovarian cysts and uterine fibroids** in females (and prostate cancer, sexual dysfunction and altered sperm in males).
- **Type 2 diabetes and its precursor, insulin resistance.**
- **Heart disease and heart rhythm abnormalities in patients.**
- **Liver disease.**
- **Thyroid dysfunction.**
- **Obesity and greater accumulation of fat in cells.**

Unborn babies, infants and children are especially susceptible to BPA's harmful effects because they are still growing. *Exposure before birth and/or during childhood has been linked to...*

- **Birth defects.**
- **Cognitive problems, including learning deficits.**
- **Behavioral problems, such as conditions involving hyperactivity.**
- **Early puberty in females.**
- **Increased risk for cancer in adulthood.**

How much is too much? The EPA estimates that exposure of up to 50 micrograms (mcg) of BPA per kilogram (kg) of body weight per day is safe. However, recent studies suggest that even a tiny fraction of this amount—as little as 0.025 mcg/kg per day—may be dangerous, especially to unborn babies, infants and children.

Dr. vom Saal said, "No matter what you might hear from the plastics industry, which is trying to convince consumers that BPA is safe, hundreds of published papers show that BPA is a toxin with no safe levels."

Scary: When the CDC studied urine samples of more than 2,500 Americans age six and older, 93% of those tested had BPA in their urine.

BPA SELF-DEFENSE

Here are Dr. vom Saal's suggestions for minimizing your exposure to BPA…

• **Avoid canned foods when possible.**

Note: It does not help to store cans in the refrigerator or to use canned goods soon after you buy them. The harm is already done even before the cans reach the market because high heat must be used to sterilize the food during canning.

Exceptions: There are several manufacturers—including Eco Fish, Eden Organic, Edward & Sons, Muir Glen, Oregon's Choice Gourmet Albacore and Wild Planet—that have begun using BPA-free cans for some of their products. (See a manufacturer's Web site for information on its BPA-free canned products, or contact the company directly.)

• **Cardboard cartons** (such as those used for juice or milk) and cardboard cylindrical "cans" (such as those used for raisins) generally are better options than metal cans—but they are not ideal because they may contain some recycled paper (which is loaded with BPA)…or they may be lined with a resin that contains BPA.

Best: Opt for foods that are fresh or frozen or that come in glass bottles or jars or in foil pouches.

• **Never give canned liquid formula to an infant.** Powdered is much safer.

• **When microwaving, never let plastic wrap come in contact with your food.** If a product has a plastic film covering that is supposed to be left in place during microwave cooking, remove the film and replace it with a glass or ceramic cover instead.

Even if the instructions on a prepackaged food say to microwave the product in the plastic pouch it comes in, you should transfer the food to a glass or ceramic container before cooking.

• **Check the triangle-enclosed recycling numeral** on plastic items that come in contact with foods or beverages—storage containers, water pitchers, baby bottles, sippy cups, utensils and tableware. The numeral "7" indicates a plastic that may or may not contain BPA. To be safe, Dr. vom Saal said, "If you see a numeral '7' and it doesn't say BPA-free, assume there is BPA." The letters "PC" stamped near the recycling number are another indication that the plastic contains BPA.

• **Recheck what's in your cupboards.** Many commonly used products like travel mugs are made from this kind of plastic.

• **Plastics labeled number two or five,** which also are often used for food containers, do not have BPA. But they may contain other potentially harmful chemicals that can leach out, especially when heat breaks down the molecular bonds of plastic. To be safe, wash all plastic kitchenware in cold to room-temperature water with a mild cleanser, not in the dishwasher. Never microwave plastic containers—not even those labeled microwave-safe, such as frozen entrée trays. Instead use a glass or ceramic container. Before putting hot soup or gravy into plastic containers to freeze, first allow it to cool. Throw out any plastic kitchenware that is scratched, chipped or discolored—damaged plastic is most likely to leach chemicals.

• **Do not assume that plastics with no triangle-enclosed numeral are safe.** Dr. vom Saal cautioned, "Manufacturers know that consumers are looking for BPA, so they're taking identifying numbers off their products and packaging." Don't fall prey to such tricks.

The Common Food Additive That Can Addle Your Brain

Suzanne de la Monte, MD, study leader and associate professor of pathology and medicine, Brown University, Providence, Rhode Island.

Bronwyn Schweigerdt, nutrition instructor and author of *Free to Eat: The Proven Recipe for Permanent Weight Loss* (Peripity). *www.fiber-girl.com.*

What if the increasingly common use of an everyday food additive and fertilizer—found in ground beef, bacon, bologna, beer and cheese...and in agricultural runoff that ends up in drinking water—was the unsuspected cause of the striking rise in the number of people with Alzheimer's disease?

That's the shocking (but well-substantiated) theory of a team of researchers from Brown University in Rhode Island, detailed in a recent issue of the *Journal of Alzheimer's Disease*.

NITRITES AND NITRATES

The researchers looked at the yearly death rates from diseases of aging, such as stroke, Alzheimer's disease (AD) and type 2 diabetes mellitus (T2DM). Then they matched those rates against exposure to nitrites (used as food additives) and nitrates (used as food additives and in fertilizer).

Result: They found a surprising parallel between increasingly high death rates from AD and increasingly high exposure to nitrites and nitrates.

Between 1968 and 2005, the death rates from AD among 75- to 84-year-olds increased 150-fold, while death rates from stroke in the same age group declined.

"These data show that trends in death rates from AD are not due to an aging population," says Suzanne de la Monte, MD, the study leader. "Such a dramatic increase in death rates in a relatively short interval of time is more consistent with exposure-related causes."

EXPOSURE TO WHAT?

As death rates from AD were skyrocketing, so was the use of nitrate-containing fertilizer, which increased by 230% between 1955 and 2005.

And between 1970 and 2005, sales from fast-food chains and meat processing companies (processed meat is a major source of nitrites and nitrates in the diet) increased by more than eightfold.

"It is conceivable that chronic exposure to relatively low levels of nitrites, nitrates and nitrosamines [formed by the body from nitrites and nitrates] through processed foods, fertilizers and water is responsible for the current epidemic of AD, and for the increasing mortality rates associated with it," says Dr. de la Monte.

Theory: "We have become a 'nitrosamine' generation, she says. "We now eat a diet rich in amines from protein, and rich in nitrites and nitrates from additives, a combination that leads to increased nitrosamine production in the body. And not only do we consume nitrites and nitrates in processed foods, but nitrates get into our food supply by leeching from the soil and contaminating water supplies used for crop irrigation, food processing and drinking."

Surprising: That increased exposure to nitrates and nitrites might not only be causing the epidemic of Alzheimer's—it might also be causing the epidemic of type 2 diabetes mellitus (T2DM).

Nitrosamines can spark biochemical factors that create the chronic low-grade inflammation and oxidation underlying both AD and T2DM, explains Dr. de la Monte.

In her research, Dr. de la Monte found that the nitrosamine-like drug *streptozotocin*—used in animal experiments to induce diabetes—also causes AD-type neurodegeneration and cognitive impairment.

And studies now show that having T2DM nearly doubles your risk of developing AD.

"In essence, at the core of the development of AD and T2DM is insulin resistance with associated deficits in glucose utilization and energy metabolism, and increased levels of chronic inflammation and oxidative stress," she says.

"The prevalence rates of these two diseases have increased sharply over the past several decades and show no sign of plateau. Because there has been a relatively short time interval for this dramatic shift in disease incidence and prevalence rates, we believe the increase is caused by environmental exposures."

MINIMIZE AND AVOID

To stop the flood of nitrites and nitrates, Dr. de la Monte advocates reforms in public health policies. "We need to eliminate the use of nitrites and nitrates in food processing, preservation and agriculture...take steps to prevent the formation of nitrosamines...and employ safe and effective means to detoxify food and water before human consumption."

But while you're waiting for industry and government to protect you from nitrates, nitrites and nitrosamines, here's how you can protect yourself...

• **Minimize or avoid foods high in nitrites.** "Just about everybody in my lab changed what they ate after the results of this study," says Dr. de la Monte. "They stopped or minimized eating foods with added nitrites and nitrates."

• **Look at the label of any processed or preserved food, she advises.** If it lists nitrites or nitrates—additives used for coloring (to make red meat redder), flavoring and as preservatives—don't buy it. "This is the easiest lifestyle change I can recommend."

Examples: processed meats (such as bacon, sausage, hot dogs and luncheon meats), cheese and cheese products, beer, nonfat dry milk.

• **Minimize or avoid cooking methods that form nitrosamines.** These include frying and flame broiling, she says.

• **Eat more fruits and vegetables.** "They help prevent the formation of nitrosamines in the stomach," says nutritionist Bronwyn Schweigerdt, in Oakland, California.

Health Food Imposters—Healthy Foods That Actually Aren't

Jonny Bowden, a board-certified nutrition specialist, a nationally known weight loss coach and author of *The 150 Healthiest Foods on Earth: The Surprising, Unbiased Truth about What You Should Eat and Why* (Fair Winds). *www.jonnybowden.com.*

The reputation of some foods seems to change as often as the weather. Foods we once shunned we now embrace as good for us—certain fats, coconut oil, whole eggs and even coffee come to mind. Then there's the flip side. The grocery store aisles now abound with foods purported to be healthy, but in fact are junk disguised in wholesome packaging.

A prime example of this from recent history is margarine. It was introduced as a healthy alternative to butter, but many margarines are actually loaded with trans fat, and may be far worse for you than the rather innocent butter it replaced. (It's possible that an exception is the plant sterol-enriched margarines recently brought to market, but we don't know enough about them yet, so the jury is still out on their health value.) And what about some of the other staples of the health-food industry? Are they really as "good" for us as we've been led to believe?

Jonny Bowden is a board certified nutritionist. *Here's what he had to say on that topic...*

BREAKFAST CEREALS AND MEAL-REPLACEMENT BARS—TOO GOOD TO BE TRUE?

The claim of many cereals to be "whole grain" is wholly misleading. Labeling laws let marketers flash "health benefits" if they are carefully worded. "The fact that something started as whole grain doesn't mean much if all the nutrition has been processed out of it," says Bowden. "Many cereal labels today say 'made from whole grains'." The truth is they're made from flours and cereals manufactured from whole grains, which raise blood sugar almost as high as other processed ones. These 'whole grain' cereals have been processed to the point where they have around 2 grams (g) or less of fiber per serving, which is minimal." In Bowden's opinion, whole grain cereals with less than 5 g of fiber per serving are no better than the cereals they replaced.

"Additionally, many cereal- and grain-based breakfast products are loaded with sugar, some have trans fat, and most also have additives," said Bowden. He advised reading the label carefully. Strive to find brands with about 10 grams of protein (or close to that), no hydrogenated oils and no more than a couple of grams of sugar per serving. This doesn't mean you have to give up this convenient food category altogether. For example, the Atkins Advantage bars meet that criteria, as do a few—very few—others. "There are also good bars that have more sugar than three grams," he added, "but those are specialty whole-foods bars, such as Omega Smart...Bumble Bars...and Lara Bars, made from nothing but real fruit, spices and nuts." All of these are healthy.

Most other energy and meal replacement bars have very high sugar and belong in the candy aisle. As they say—"if it's too good to be true, it probably is!"

OY, SOY TOO

Soy has been a health darling of recent years, to the extent that it has become the primary source of protein in many protein-enriched products. However, the bloom is off that rose. "I don't think soy is the worst thing in the world for you," Bowden said, "but I think it's been way oversold as a health food." The healthy kind of soy is that which is traditionally fermented, like miso and tempeh, or minimally processed, like edamame. "Those are the soy products that have real health benefits," says Bowden, adding that other soy products (such as many meal-replacement bars) should be enjoyed in moderation.

SOMETHING FISHY ABOUT SALMON

"Farm-raised salmon is another problem," said Bowden. "Nutritionists have long urged everyone to eat salmon for its high content of omega-3s and because it's such a wonderful source of protein and vitamins. But that is not actually true of farm-raised salmon (versus wild salmon), which encompasses most of the Atlantic salmon we eat. These fish are farm raised, kept in pens, fed antibiotics, artificially colored and often contain far fewer omega-3s than their wild cousins." Bowden suggests looking for wild Alaskan salmon, which is preferable to the farm-raised kind. "If you can't get it in the supermarket, try a company like Vital Choice (*www.vitalchoice.com*, 800-608-4825), which will ship the highest quality wild salmon and other fish directly to your door," he says.

A good rule of thumb: The colder the water the fish lives in, the more omega-3s it will likely have.

CANOLA OIL: NO CAN DO

Neither is Bowden a fan of canola oil. "The presence of canola oil in the marketplace is a triumph of marketing over science," he told me. "Canola oil is a highly processed oil that needs to be deodorized at high temperatures, which frequently creates trans fat," he said. "In addition, the omega-3s in it are easily damaged by heating." If you want to use canola oil, stick to cold-pressed organic canola oil and use it for dressings, but not for cooking.

YOGURT

Most of us have already figured out that yogurt—a major health craze a couple of decades ago—is not all that healthy in the drinkable and squeezable and high-sugar forms that are available today. What about frozen yogurt? "Its only resemblance to real yogurt is that they're both white," Bowden said. "Seriously, it can be a delicious dessert, but don't fool yourself that frozen yogurt is healthier than ice cream. In fact, the nonfat kind is often filled with aspartame, which can be a problem for many people," he said. You might as well eat the highest-quality ice cream you can find. "Just eat it less often," he suggested.

FRUIT DRINKS

Another great pretender? Commercial fruit beverages, especially many of the kinds marketed and conveniently packaged for kids' lunches, are nothing but sugar water. "You are far better off drinking water and flavoring it with lemon or cherry or berry juice concentrate, which are high in antioxidants. Or, if you really want the juice, dilute it with water in a 1:4, solution so you take in less sugar," Bowden said. Healthy exceptions to the "no juice" rule are 100% juices made from cranberry and pomegranate, which do, in fact, contain plenty of important and desirable nutrients. If you don't mind paying a premium, you can also choose from an ever-growing selection of "healthy" juices sold in specialty and health food stores, made of better ingredients (organic and with less or no added sugar, chemicals or "fruit juice fillers").

It's easy to be fooled by the advertising claims made for many products. Be skeptical, and smart. "The healthiest foods are the ones that are minimally processed and closest to the state in which they were found in nature. If you could hunt it, fish for it, pluck it or gather it, chances are it's the real thing, not a health-food imposter."

Don't Fall for the Hype Of "Functional Foods"

Rebecca Shannonhouse, editor, *Bottom Line/Health* newsletter, 281 Tresser Boulevard, Stamford, Connecticut 06901.

Supermarket shelves are now filled with "functional foods"—products designed to provide health benefits beyond the food's basic nutritional value.

Examples: A new version of Tropicana orange juice contains 3 grams (g) of fiber per serving...a spread called Benecol contains cholesterol-lowering plant *stanols*...and a yogurt called Activia contains a strain of beneficial bacteria that helps promote regular bowel movements.

Some cereals, breads and other staples have been fortified with vitamins and minerals for decades. But the new functional foods have some nutrition experts worried.

"People who start adding foods to their diets because they're 'good for them' could end up consuming more calories if they do not eliminate other foods," says Alice H. Lichtenstein, DSc, professor of nutrition sciences at Tufts University in Boston. The health risks from obesity could far outweigh any of the likely benefits, she explains.

Other potential drawbacks...

- **Foods that are clearly bad for people**, such as soft drinks, could be marketed as "healthy," once they're spiked with vitamin C, calcium or other nutrients.
- **Foods can be less reliable** and/or less convenient than supplements for getting some substances, such as plant stanols.

Even though functional foods may be tempting to try, you're better off following the tried-and-true nutritional advice we all grew up with: Eat a diet rich in vegetables, fruits and whole grains...include cold-water fish, such as salmon or mackerel, two times per week...and balance the calories you eat with those you burn.

Short on Omega-3s

Foods with added omega-3s often contain little or none of the types of omega-3s that are best for the heart. The omega-3s *docosahexaenoic acid* (DHA) and *eicosapentaenoic acid* (EPA) are far more prevalent in fish than in other sources. Six ounces of farmed Atlantic salmon provides about 3,500 milligrams (mg) of DHA and EPA...six ounces of sardines, about 3,000 mg. Foods supplemented with omega-3s provide much less—one Land O'Lakes Omega-3 egg, 350 mg...one cup of Silk Plus Omega-3 DHA Soy Milk, 32 mg.

Best: Get omega-3s from fish, such as salmon, sardines, mackerel and herring.

Katherine Talmadge, registered dietitian, Washington, DC, and spokesperson, American Dietetic Association, Washington, DC.

Foods That Seem Healthy...But Really Are Not

David Grotto, RD, president and founder of Nutrition Housecall, LLC, a consulting firm specializing in family nutrition programs, Chicago. He serves on the scientific advisory board of Men's Health magazine and is author of *101 Optimal Life Foods* (Bantam). He is past spokesman for the American Dietetic Association.

Nearly everyone wants to eat healthier. The food industry, which keeps a close eye on America's changing tastes, has introduced thousands of foods that purport to be healthy—but are they really?

Too many people assume that anything that comes from a health-food store is good for you or that quantities don't matter when you're eating a "good" food.

Personal story: One of my first clients was a strict vegetarian, but this woman was 5'2" and weighed 250 pounds. Something was clearly amiss. She told me that she used nearly a pint of olive oil in recipes because it's a "healthy" fat.

Some foods, such as vegetables, whole grains, legumes, etc., are almost always good for you. But many of the foods that are promoted with healthy-sounding terms, such as "natural" or "vitamin-packed," actually are loaded with sugar and/or fat and are unacceptably high in calories.

Some common offenders—and healthier alternatives…

• **Smoothies.** Some smoothies can have more calories than sodas, making them an unhealthy choice to have regularly. My daughter once bought a peanut butter smoothie. I did the calculations and found that it had about 1,000 calories.

Healthier: Make your own smoothie using just fresh fruit and adding skim milk if you want. Or mix four ounces of fruit juice with four ounces of sparkling water. It tastes delicious, is relatively low in calories and has the same nutrients as a serving of whole fruit (though less fiber).

• **Protein bars.** Millions of Americans replace one or more meals daily with bars—granola bars, high-protein bars, meal-replacement bars, etc. Many of these are high in sugar and/or fat and deliver 300 calories or more. It's fine to occasionally use one of these bars as a meal replacement, but they're too high in calories to have in addition to meals.

Healthier: Make up your own healthy snacks, using a mixture of nuts, seeds and dried fruit. One-half ounce of almonds (about 12) and one tablespoon of dried fruit totals about 140 calories. When you do crave a bar, have one that has at least three grams of fiber, with no more than 150 calories. Try Luna small-size organic bars.

• **Frozen yogurt.** Healthier than ice cream? Not necessarily. Yogurt is one of the healthiest foods you can eat, but most frozen brands have more in common with desserts than with health foods.

Check the label: Some frozen yogurts have the same number of calories as ice cream. They may even have similar amounts of sugar and fat. Also, it's rare to find live and active cultures—the organisms that make natural yogurt so healthy—in frozen products.

Healthier: One of the newer versions of frozen yogurt. For example, Forever Yogurt, a yogurt chain based in Chicago, is producing products that are relatively low in fat and sugar and contain live and active cultures. Other manufacturers are following suit, such as New England–based Brigham's with its premium frozen yogurt, élan. Look for the LAC seal on frozen yogurt containers—it means that the product has at least 10 million live and active cultures.

• **Pretzels.** They're often touted as a healthier alternative to potato chips because they have less fat. A one-ounce pretzel serving usually has about one gram of fat, compared to up to 10 grams in a one-ounce serving of some potato chips. However, most pretzels are high in salt. They also have a high glycemic index because they consist mostly of refined wheat flour and cornstarch—they're quickly transformed to sugar during digestion, which can increase blood glucose levels and lead to weight gain.

Be wary of pretzels with added wheat or oat bran—these often are just "window dressing" and not a significant source of whole grains.

Healthier: Satisfy your "crunch craving" with a mix of nuts, seeds and dried fruit (see under "protein bars" mentioned earlier).

• **Fake whole-wheat bread.** Real whole-wheat bread is among the healthiest foods you can eat. Some brands, however, only look like whole wheat—manufacturers have been known to add a brown color to make them look more wholesome.

Another trick: Manufacturers super-size the slices so that they can make higher fiber claims on the label.

Healthier: A bread with normal-size slices that contains at least three grams of fiber per serving. Read the ingredient label. The word "whole"—whole wheat, whole grain, etc.—should be first in the list.

• **Muffins.** Today's big muffins often seem like they're loaded with nutritious ingredients, such as fruit or bran, but many muffins that are sold in supermarkets or coffee shops, such as Starbucks, are loaded with fat and sugar and range from 400 to 500 calories each.

Healthier: A small one-and-a-half ounce muffin that's made with bran or a whole grain.

A muffin this size that's not loaded with sugar and/or fat usually contains about 100 calories.

• **Rice mixes.** Brown rice has more fiber and disease-fighting phytochemicals than white rice, but people don't always want to take the time to cook brown rice. Instead, they buy a packaged rice pilaf, both for convenience and extra flavor. Most of these products are very high in sodium, as well as fat.

Healthier: Uncle Ben's microwavable brown rice. It's ready in just a few minutes, and you can season it to your own taste—without adding salt or oil.

fructose, the component that is considered to have potentially adverse effects," explains Dr. Havel. "Results from studies comparing both types of sugar suggest that overconsumption of either could lead to higher levels of fats in the blood, known as triglycerides, and possibly weight gain."

Americans consume an average of about 85 pounds of sweeteners—both HFCS and white sugar—a year. We would all do better if we limited our consumption of foods made with any added sugar.

Foods That Aren't So Nutritious After All

Rebecca Shannonhouse, editor, *Bottom Line/Health* newsletter, 281 Tresser Boulevard, Stamford, Connecticut 06901.

If a food label touts its product as "100% natural" or "100% whole grain," you might assume that all the ingredients are nutritious. But that's not always the case.

For instance, it's no surprise to find the sweetener high-fructose corn syrup (HFCS) in super-sweet sodas, but many people are shocked to learn that it is also found in many food products that are promoted as healthful.

Examples: Some whole-grain breads and cereals, granola bars, yogurts, "low-fat, low-cholesterol" cookies and many brands of fruit juice. Manufacturers often use HFCS because it is usually cheaper than sugar.

Some scientists have speculated that HFCS (derived from corn) may have different biological effects than regular sugar (derived from sugarcane or sugar beets), making it more likely to cause diabetes, obesity and other health problems.

While there are real concerns about HFCS, there's no conclusive evidence at this point that it is worse than table sugar (sucrose), says Peter J. Havel, PhD, a nutrition researcher at the University of California, Davis. "Both table sugar and HFCS contain similar amounts of

Chocolate Is Not a Health Food

Like red wine, fruits and vegetables, cocoa contains flavonoids, antioxidants that may reduce the risk for coronary artery disease—but most flavonoids are removed when the cocoa is processed and made into chocolate. Also, the added sugar and fat make chocolate—even chocolate that is marketed as good for you—a nutritional loser.

Best: If you like the flavor of chocolate, enjoy it sparingly.

Suzanne Havala Hobbs, DrPH, RD, clinical associate professor, department of health policy and administration, University of North Carolina, Chapel Hill.

Organic Junk Food

Rebecca Shannonhouse, editor, *Bottom Line/Health* newsletter, 281 Tresser Boulevard, Stamford, Connecticut 06901.

Natural food stores and supermarkets now are giving more and more shelf space to "organic" snacks, such as potato chips, ice cream and cookies.

But is organic junk food more healthful? Not necessarily. You'll often see the same list of potentially unhealthful ingredients on organic product labels as you will on conventional snack labels. For example, organic chips (which are made with organically grown potatoes) can still be loaded with sodium, and they will drive up blood pressure just as efficiently as conventional chips.

According to Sandra Woodruff, a Tallahassee, Florida–based registered dietitian and the author of *The Complete Diabetes Prevention Plan* (Avery), organic junk food is still junk food. A pint of super-premium organic ice cream can have 1,000 to 1,200 calories and more saturated fat than you should eat in two days. That's no better than super-rich nonorganic snacks.

The US Department of Agriculture has stringent rules for the use of the word "organic"—food manufacturers are not allowed to use most conventional pesticides or synthetic fertilizers...antibiotics...or growth hormones—but those rules don't necessarily mean that the product is healthful.

Read the label: If a food is high in sodium, saturated fat or sugar, limit your intake.

Better: Choose organics that list wholesome, minimally processed ingredients, such as cookies made with whole-grain flour rather than white flour...or a snack made with liquid vegetable oil instead of a saturated fat, such as palm kernel oil.

It's up to you to know that the organic label doesn't always tell the whole story.

SPECIAL REPORT #2

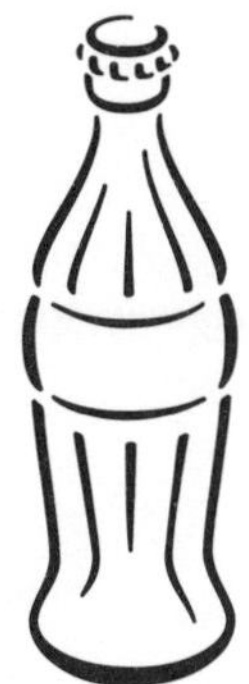

Food Lies & Dirty Labeling Tricks

Food Lies & Dirty Labeling Tricks

The Truth About Dairy Foods

Most Americans grew up believing that dairy foods are synonymous with strong bones and good health. Many of my patients proudly tell me that they always have a glass of milk with dinner. These days, the dairy industry spends a fortune promoting milk as a healthful food. At the same time, many health experts suggest that dairy consumption (chiefly milk, yogurt, cheese, butter and ice cream) may lead to health problems. What's the truth?

Most people believe that dairy foods help prevent osteoporosis. Not so, according to the landmark Harvard Nurses' Health Study. In this study, scientists followed more than 77,000 women for 12 years to examine the possible link between calcium-rich foods, including milk, and osteoporosis. The researchers found no evidence that drinking milk prevents this bone-thinning disease. Some plant sources of calcium are more readily absorbed by the body and more likely to support healthy bone cells.

Example: Sesame butter is a good calcium source and is delicious on toast or rice crackers. Leafy, green vegetables are high in calcium, too. For example, one cup of cooked collard greens contains 266 milligrams (mg) of calcium.

There's also widespread confusion related to dairy's impact on heart disease. Whole-fat versions of dairy products are high in saturated fats, which increase the risk for cardiovascular disease. Studies also have linked dairy consumption to an increased risk for prostate cancer. Nonorganic dairy of any sort increases your exposure to toxins and hormones, which are thought to increase cancer risk.

When it comes to dairy, people can be lactose intolerant (the inability to digest dairy

Jamison Starbuck, ND, is a naturopathic physician in family practice in Missoula, Montana. She is past president of the American Association of Naturopathic Physicians and a contributing editor to *The Alternative Advisor: The Complete Guide to Natural Therapies and Alternative Treatments* (Time Life).

sugar) or they can be allergic to the proteins in dairy. When lactose intolerant people eat dairy, they suffer from indigestion, gas and irritable bowel symptoms.

People with a dairy allergy suffer from more than just bowel symptoms when they eat dairy. Allergic reactions cause inflammation throughout the body, most notably in the upper respiratory tract. Dairy allergy is a common cause of frequent sinusitis, ear infection and repeated colds.

Dairy foods do not promote disease as readily as soda, fried foods or candy, but it's clear that dairy can trigger some health problems. That's why I tell my patients to seek healthful alternatives to dairy. Vegetables, nuts, seeds, legumes and whole grains are excellent sources of essential minerals, such as calcium, magnesium and zinc. Avocado, olive oil, sesame oil and fish are more healthful sources of fat than cheese or whole milk.

My advice: If you don't have high cholesterol (LDL "bad" cholesterol above 129 mg/dL in those who are not at risk for heart disease) and you are not allergic to dairy, enjoy small amounts as you would chocolate, wine or red meat. It's fine to sprinkle Parmesan cheese on a salad, have a slice of cheese on a sandwich or enjoy a cup of yogurt. Just watch your reactions to dairy and don't be taken in by the marketing hype. Some people may need a calcium supplement. Discuss this with your doctor.

Sneaky Trans Fats—They Harm More Than Your Heart

JoAnn E. Manson, MD, DrPH, a professor of medicine and women's health at Harvard Medical School and chief of the division of preventive medicine at Brigham and Women's Hospital, both in Boston. A lead investigator for two highly influential studies on women's health, Dr. Manson is coauthor of *Hot Flashes, Hormones & Your Health* (McGraw-Hill).

No doubt you've heard warnings about trans fats. But are you really sure what they are, why they are bad for you—and how to avoid them? *Here's what you need to know...*

• Trans fats are "fake" fats. Some meats and dairy products contain small amounts of naturally occurring trans fats—but 80% of trans fats are artificially produced. Trans fats are created by adding hydrogen to liquid vegetable oils to make them more solid. The purpose of these fake fats is to give foods texture and extend shelf life.

• Even small amounts harm your heart. Getting just 1% to 3% of your daily calories from trans fats—about 2 gram (g) to 6 g, or the amount that could be found in a slice of pie—increases your risk for cardiovascular problems. Trans fats raise LDL "bad" cholesterol...lower HDL "good" cholesterol...increase inflammation...and interfere with artery wall function.

New evidence: In four studies involving nearly 140,000 participants, a mere 2% increase in calorie intake from trans fats was linked to a 23% increased risk for heart disease. The Nurses' Health Study measured trans fats in women's red blood cells and found that women in the highest 25% were more than three times as likely to develop heart problems as those in the lowest 25%.

• The impact on health may be wide-ranging. Trans fats appear more likely than other fats to promote weight gain. They have been linked to the development of diabetes, especially in people who are overweight, inactive or otherwise predisposed to the disease. Trans fats also may boost the risk for infertility, cancer and Alzheimer's disease.

• Trans fats lurk in unsuspected foods. You may know that trans fats are found in many deep-fried fast foods (french fries, onion rings), commercially baked goods (doughnuts, cookies), packaged snacks (chips, crackers), shortening and some margarines. But even supposedly "good-for-you" foods—such as soup and microwave popcorn—sometimes have trans fats. And did you realize that some foods claiming to have zero trans fats still contain these bad fats?

Reason: Nutrition labels can list a trans fat content of zero if a single serving has less than

0.5 grams of trans fat—even if a "suggested serving size" is unrealistically small compared with what people usually eat (for instance, one-third of a muffin). *Self-defense...*

- **In the supermarket**—if the ingredients list includes the phrase "partially hydrogenated vegetable oil," the food contains trans fats...so skip it.
- **In restaurants**—avoid the foods listed above unless the manager confirms that the food is trans fat–free.

Junk-Food Ads Trigger More Eating

Adults watched a TV show with commercials that showed unhealthful foods (candy, cola)...or more healthful fare (oatmeal, orange juice)...or no food.

Later: TV off, participants were offered snacks. Those who had watched junk-food ads ate significantly more overall than the others.

Lesson: Turn off the TV or leave the room during junk-food ads.

Jennifer Harris, PhD, director of marketing initiatives, Rudd Center for Food Policy and Obesity, Yale University, New Haven, Connecticut, and leader of a study of 98 adults.

How Food Labels Legally Lie

Suzanne Havala Hobbs, DrPh, RD, clinical assistant professor, School of Public Health, University of North Carolina at Chapel Hill. She is author of *The Natural Kitchen: The Complete Guide to Buying and Using Natural Foods and Products*. (Berkley). Environmental Working Group. *www.ewg.org.*

If you are confused about the claims that manufacturers are now making on food labels, you are not alone.

"ORGANIC"

The term organic is hotly debated. The US Department of Agriculture's (USDA) current definition states that organic foods are those plants produced without the use of pesticides, sewage sludge (for fertilization) or synthetic fertilizer...or those animals raised without hormones or antibiotics.

To read more about it, go to the USDA's Web site at *www.ams.usda.gov* and click on "National Organic Program."

Organic foods, including produce, meat and dairy products, typically cost more than nonorganic varieties.

The FDA has linked pesticides to some types of cancer. Other studies have linked them to Parkinson's disease. There's also strong evidence from the American Medical Association that bacteria are becoming resistant to some antibiotics because they are used in the process of meat production.

What you can do: Whenever possible, buy organic meats and dairy products.

What you may not know: In October 2005, the Agricultural Appropriations Conference Committee voted to allow synthetic ingredients into foods labeled "organic." Therefore, yogurt, pudding and other items may be considered organic even if they contain synthetic additives.

For produce, choose organic varieties if you're buying one of the items found by the Environmental Working Group (a nonprofit group of researchers who investigate environmental health threats) to be among the most contaminated (see next page).

If you must buy nonorganic, choose produce that is least likely to be contaminated. Wash the nonorganic produce vigorously under running water to remove as much potentially harmful residue as possible. (Organic produce also should be washed.)

If you must buy nonorganic meat, choose the leanest cuts available and, whenever possible, remove the skin from poultry (toxins from hormones and antibiotics tend to accumulate in fatty tissue).

"NATURAL"

"Natural"—used for marketing purposes—it is not a term that is defined by the government.

What you may not know: Natural does not mean that a food product is "healthful."

Example: Breyers labels its ice cream "all natural," but it is high in fat and saturated fat.

What you can do: Read food labels carefully to determine the levels of fat and saturated fat as well as other ingredients in products that are labeled natural.

"LOW"

Many dairy products and some processed foods, such as soup, frozen entrees and snacks, use the term "low" or some variation thereof. *What these terms mean...*

Low fat: 3 grams (g) or less of total fat per serving.

Low saturated fat: 1 g or less of saturated fat per serving.

Low calorie: 40 calories or less per serving.

Low cholesterol: 20 milligrams (mg) or less of cholesterol and 2 g or less of saturated fat per serving.

Low sodium: 140 mg or less of sodium per serving.

Very low sodium: 35 mg or less of sodium per serving.

Nonfat: Less than 0.5 g of fat per serving.

"LEAN" AND "EXTRA-LEAN"

"Lean" and "extra-lean" refers to the fat content of meat, poultry and seafood. *What these two terms mean...*

Lean: Less than 10 g of fat, including no more than 4 g of saturated fat and less than 95 mg of cholesterol per 3.5-ounce serving.

Extra-lean: Less than 5 g of fat, including no more than 2 g of saturated fat and less than 95 mg of cholesterol per 3.5-ounce serving.

OTHER TERMS

Reduced: Contains at least 25% less of an ingredient (such as fat, cholesterol, sodium or sugar) or calories than the regular product.

Example: Reduced Fat Fig Newtons have at least 25% less fat than the original recipe.

High: Contains at least 20% of the Daily Value (recommended daily intake) for a particular nutrient.

Example: The Daily Value for fiber is 25 g. If a food product contains 5 g of fiber per serving, it might say "high fiber" on its label.

WHEN ORGANIC IS WORTH THE PRICE

Most Contaminated Produce
(Best to buy organic)

Apples	Peaches
Bell peppers	Pears
Celery	Potatoes
Cherries	Red raspberries
Imported grapes	Spinach
Nectarines	Strawberries

LEAST CONTAMINATED PRODUCE
(Ok to buy nonorganic)

Asparagus	Kiwi
Avocados	Mangoes
Bananas	Onions
Broccoli	Papaya
Cauliflower	Peas (sweet)
Corn (sweet)	Pineapples

More Ways to Decipher Food Labels

Suzanne Havala Hobbs, DrPh, RD, clinical assistant professor, School of Public Health, University of North Carolina at Chapel Hill. She is author of *The Natural Kitchen: The Complete Guide to Buying and Using Natural Foods and Products.* (Berkley). Environmental Working Group. *www.ewg.org.*

The claims made on food labels can't always be taken at face value. There are rules that govern how certain words can be used on food packaging, but these rules often leave room for deception. Food companies eager to sell their products take full advantage of these loopholes.

Among the most potentially confusing food label terms...

• **Free range.** Some people feel better about eating eggs or poultry that come from "free range" birds. They imagine these birds living relatively normal lives, not confined to pens. Unfortunately, this might not be the case.

According to the US Department of Agriculture (USDA), poultry can be labeled "free range" as long as outdoor access was made available to the bird "for an undetermined period each day." A single door to a large coop might have been opened for a few minutes, with only a small percentage of the birds making the dash outside.

There's no USDA definition at all for the term "free range" when it comes to eggs. It's possible that the bird that laid your "free range" eggs never saw the light of day.

• **Fresh.** The word "fresh" often means exactly what it seems to—that a food has not been frozen, heated or chemically preserved. But when the word is used as part of the phrase "fresh-baked," the only guarantee is that it is fresh until the sell-by date.

When "fresh" is used as part of the phrase "fresh frozen," not only has the food been frozen, it might have been blanched—quickly scalded—as well. Blanching deactivates enzymes in vegetables that might otherwise cause loss of color, flavor and texture.

• **Light.** Very specific rules govern the terms "light" and "lite." In general, the food must be reduced in calories by one-third or have half the fat or sodium. "Light" potato chips have 50% less fat than regular chips. Food makers also are allowed to use this word to describe foods that are light in other ways—a fruitcake labeled "light" simply might have been made with white sugar rather than brown sugar. The product's label must then state which attribute "light" is referring to—for example, "light in color" or "light in texture."

• **Serving size.** Many consumers overlook the fact that nutritional data on food labels is in per-serving terms. A large cookie might be labeled "200 calories" or "10 grams of fat" per serving—but if the label shows the cookie is equal to two servings, the calorie and fat contents in the whole cookie are actually double that amount.

• **No trans fat.** Government regulations now require most food manufacturers to list the number of grams of trans fat in packaged foods on the packaging. Trans fats, often listed as "partially hydrogenated vegetable oil," can increase your risk of heart disease by increasing your total and LDL ("bad") cholesterol.

Label loophole: If the trans fat totals less than one-half gram per serving and no label claims are made about fat, fatty acids or cholesterol, trans fat information doesn't have to be listed. Even if trans fat is included in the product, if the amount totals less than one-half gram per serving, manufacturers can list the amount as zero and advertise the food as having no trans fat. Eating several servings could result in an intake of a few grams of trans fat.

SPECIAL REPORT #3

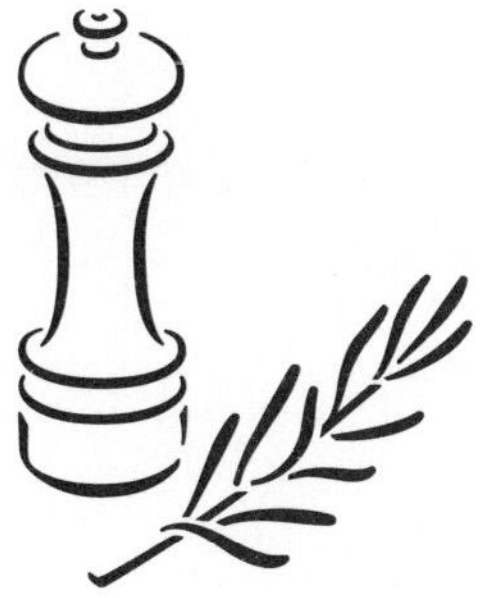

Best-Ever Healing Herbs & Spices

Best-Ever Healing Herbs & Spices

The Medicine in Your Spice Rack

Many herbs and spices do more than simply flavor food. Research suggests that certain seasonings help prevent or relieve various medical conditions. For general health, the herbs and spices below can be stirred into food or sprinkled over it. You also can try traditional kitchen remedies or consider supplements.*

CAYENNE

Potential benefits...

- **Gas and indigestion relief.**
- **Headache relief.**
- **Circulation improvement.**

Kitchen remedies: For gas or headache—pour 1 cup boiling water over ½ teaspoon cayenne powder and stir. Drink three times daily.

Studies suggest: For cardiovascular health—30 milligrams (mg) to 120 mg of cayenne in capsule form twice daily.

CINNAMON

Potential benefits...

- **Stomach pain relief.**
- **Cholesterol reduction.**
- **Blood sugar reduction in patients with type 2 diabetes.**

Kitchen remedies: For an upset stomach—mix ¼ teaspoon ground cinnamon into 1 cup applesauce.

Studies suggest: For better blood sugar control—1,000 mg of cinnamon extract daily for six weeks.

*Some herbs and spices can interact with drugs or cause allergic reactions. Consult your doctor before using, especially if you have heart disease, diabetes, ulcers, gallstones, a bleeding or seizure disorder, a kidney or liver disorder or other health problem, or are pregnant or breast-feeding.

Catherine Ulbricht, PharmD, cofounder of the Natural Standard (*www.naturalstandard.com*), a research collaboration of information on complementary and alternative therapies. She is also chief editor of the *Journal of Dietary Supplements* and the *Journal of Herbal Pharmacotherapy.*

CLOVE

Potential benefits...

- **Anti-inflammation and sanitizing.**
- **Dental pain relief.**

Kitchen remedies: For general good health—pour 1 cup boiling water over 1 teaspoon whole cloves...steep 10 minutes...strain and drink.

Studies suggest: For dental pain—a pinch of ground clove mixed with an equal amount of glycerin (sold at health-food stores) and applied to the sore area for four minutes.

GARLIC

Potential benefits...

- **Cholesterol reduction.**
- **Blood pressure reduction.**
- **Gastric cancer risk reduction.**

Kitchen remedies: For maximum health benefits—crush fresh garlic cloves and then cook lightly...rub diced garlic onto meat before grilling to reduce carcinogens.

Studies suggest: For heart health—600 mg to 900 mg daily of noncoated garlic powder standardized to 1.3% *allicin* content, in three divided doses.**

GINGER

Potential benefits...

- **Nausea relief.**
- **Digestive improvement.**
- **Anti-inflammation.**
- **Blood clot risk reduction.**

Kitchen remedies: For nausea—pour 1 cup boiling water over ¼ teaspoon ground fresh ginger...steep 10 minutes...strain and drink.

Studies suggest: For inflammation—1 gram (g) to 4 g daily in capsule or powder form, in divided doses.**

TURMERIC

Potential benefits...

- **Alzheimer's and cancer risk reduction.**
- **Arthritis pain relief.**
- **Anti-inflammation.**

Kitchen remedies: For joint pain—steep 1 cup boiling water and ¼ teaspoon ground turmeric 15 minutes...strain and drink twice daily.

Studies suggest: For indigestion—250 mg of turmeric powder four times daily for a week.**

**Discontinue two weeks before any surgery.

Comfort in a Cup: Healing Herbal Teas

Brigitte Mars, adjunct professor of herbal medicine at Naropa University in Boulder, Colorado. She is a professional member of the American Herbalists Guild, host of the radio show *Naturally* and author of *Healing Herbal Teas* (Basic Health). *www.brigittemars.com.*

Herbal teas help soothe pain, ease stress and treat disease—more economically and with fewer side effects than drugs.

For convenience: Use tea bags.

For potency: Use loose organic herbs (sold in health-food stores).

Instructions: Boil eight ounces of water. Remove from heat. Stir in one heaping tablespoon of dried herbs or three level tablespoons of fresh herbs. Steep 10 minutes. Remove tea bag or strain off loose herbs. Drink hot or iced. Have two to three cups daily until symptoms subside...then one cup every few days to maintain health.*

- **Chamomile tea eases...**
  - Insomnia.
  - Gastrointestinal upset.
  - Inflammation.

How it works: It has mild sedative properties to calm nerves...stimulates production of digestive fluids...and may inhibit metabolism of arachidonic acid, an inflammatory omega-6 fatty acid.

Keep in mind: Steep no longer than three to five minutes to prevent bitterness. Discontinue two weeks before any surgery. Do not use if you are allergic to ragweed, celery or onion or take blood-thinning drugs.**

- **Ginger tea eases...**
  - Nausea, motion sickness and morning sickness.
  - Colds and flu.
  - Pain (sore throat, arthritis, migraine).

*Some herbs can interact with drugs or cause allergic reactions. Always consult your doctor before using herbal tea, especially if you have heart disease, diabetes, ulcers, gallbladder problems, a bleeding or seizure disorder, or a kidney or liver disorder, or if you are anticipating surgery.

How it works: It stimulates secretion of digestive fluids...reduces congestion and inflammation...and bolsters the immune system. It also reduces risk for blood clots.

Keep in mind: Steep it in hot (but not boiling) water. Discontinue two weeks before any surgery. Do not use if you have heartburn, ulcers or gallbladder problems or take blood-thinning or diabetes drugs.

- **Ginseng tea eases...**
  - Low energy.
  - Low libido.

How it works: It boosts the immune system...increases the body's resistance to stress...and contains phytosterols (steroid-like plant chemicals) that may promote proper hormone function.

Keep in mind: For best effect, drink between meals. Discontinue two weeks before any surgery. Do not use if you take blood-thinning or diabetes medication...or have a history of breast cancer.**

- **Nettle tea eases...**
  - Arthritis pain.
  - Bloating.
  - Allergies, asthma.

How it works: It reduces inflammation...acts as a diuretic...and may deactivate mast cells (which release histamine, a chemical that provokes mucous membrane hyperactivity).

Keep in mind: It is best to use dried nettle—the fresh plant can cause a stinging rash. Discontinue if it causes gastrointestinal upset. Do not use if you have any problems with blood sugar.**

- **Passionflower tea eases...**
  - Anxiety.
  - Stress.
  - Drug or alcohol withdrawal.

How it works: It may slow the breakdown of calming neurotransmitters...and it has sedative effects.

Keep in mind: It is slightly bitter, so add honey or agave nectar for a sweeter taste. Do not use with blood-thinning drugs or with sedating medication (sleeping pills, certain antihistamines, or painkillers).**

- **Peppermint tea eases...**
  - Stomach upset
  - Bad breath

How it works: It increases circulation to the digestive tract...improves flow of digestive fluids...calms intestinal spasms...suppresses mouth chemicals that contribute to bad breath.

Keep in mind: It is safe to use when pregnant or breast-feeding. Do not use if you have a hiatal hernia or gallbladder problems.

**Do not use if you are pregnant or breast-feeding.

Popular Herbs with Unexpected Health Benefits

Holly Phaneuf, PhD, expert in medicinal chemistry and author of *Herbs Demystified* (DaCapo). She is a member of the American Chemical Society and is currently conducting research on exercise and herb use.

You may know that the tiny, fiber-rich seeds of the flax plant can be used as a laxative and that ginger helps ease nausea. But can you name the other health benefits provided by these plant-derived remedies?

Few people can. However, credible scientific evidence shows that many herbs that are well-known for treating a particular ailment have other important—but little-known—uses.* *For example...*

ARTICHOKE LEAF

Artichoke leaf extract is used by some people with mildly elevated cholesterol levels as an alternative to prescription statin drugs. Exactly how the herb works is unknown, but animal studies suggest that it inhibits *HMG*

*If you use prescription drugs and/or have a chronic medical condition, such as diabetes, cancer or heart disease, speak to your doctor before trying herbal remedies. In some cases, herbs may interfere with medication or cause an undesired effect on a chronic medical problem. Women who are pregnant or breast-feeding also should consult a doctor before taking herbs.

CoA-reductase, an enzyme that plays a key role in the liver's production of cholesterol.

In a placebo-controlled, randomized study conducted at the University of Reading in England, adults who took 1,280 milligrams (mg) of artichoke leaf extract daily for three months reduced their cholesterol levels by 4.2%, on average, while levels increased by 1.9%, on average, in those taking a placebo.

What else artichoke leaf can do: calm indigestion. In a placebo-controlled, randomized study, patients rated their chronic indigestion as significantly improved after taking artichoke leaf extract twice daily for six weeks. Tests on rats suggest that the herb stimulates the gallbladder's production of bile, which helps facilitate the digestion of dietary fat.

Typical dose: About 320 mg daily of artichoke leaf soothes digestive complaints. This dosage can be taken until the indigestion is no longer a problem.

Caution: Avoid artichoke if you are allergic to plants in the daisy family or if you have gallstones (artichoke appears to make the gallbladder contract).

FLAX

Often used as a gentle laxative, the seed of the flax plant (flaxseed) contains fiber and phytonutrients known as *lignans*—a combination that helps draw water into the gut to speed digestion. For laxative effects, eat one tablespoon of whole or ground seeds (sprinkled on cereal, for example) daily. Be sure to drink at least eight ounces of water when eating flaxseeds to prevent them from forming a temporary blockage in the intestines.

What else flaxseed can do: help prevent breast and prostate cancers. Lignans form estrogen-like compounds that inhibit the body's production of the hormone in women and men. This effect is believed to reduce risk for estrogen-dependent malignancies, including some breast and prostate cancers.

Typical initial dose: One to two tablespoons of ground flaxseed daily, which can be increased gradually to as many as five tablespoons daily.

Grinding flaxseed (in a coffee grinder, for example) rather than eating it whole releases more of its cancer-fighting compounds. Also, ground flaxseed is better than flaxseed oil, which lacks the plant's beneficial lignans unless they are replaced during the manufacturing process.

Helpful: Be sure to refrigerate flaxseed to prolong freshness and preserve potency.

Caution: Do not consume flaxseed within two hours of taking an oral medication—flaxseed may interfere with absorption of the drug.

GARLIC

With its powerful blood-thinning effects, garlic is widely used to help prevent artery-blocking blood clots that can lead to a heart attack or stroke. The typical recommendation for this purpose is one clove of fresh garlic or one-half to three-quarters of a teaspoon of garlic powder daily.

What else garlic can do: help prevent stomach and colorectal cancers. The National Cancer Institute funded an analysis of 23 clinical studies that linked garlic consumption (raw, cooked or from garlic supplements) to a 10% to 50% decrease in risk for these types of cancers. This cancer-fighting effect is believed to result from the antioxidant activity of garlic's sulfur-containing molecules. Garlic also is a popular remedy to stave off the common cold, but research on its virus-fighting properties has shown mixed results.

Recommended: A fresh crushed garlic clove four to seven times a week.

GINGER

Ginger is widely used to treat nausea, including that due to motion sickness (one-quarter to one-half teaspoon of ginger powder)...and chemotherapy (one to two teaspoons daily of ginger powder). Ginger is believed to quell queasiness by stopping intense stomach motions that can interfere with digestion.

What else ginger can do: relieve arthritis pain. With its aspirin-like effects, ginger inhibits both *COX-1* and *COX-2* enzymes, substances that are involved in the production of inflammatory hormones known as prostaglandins.

Typical dose: One-quarter to one-half teaspoon daily of ginger powder.

TURMERIC

In India, turmeric is a popular remedy for indigestion. It contains *curcumin*, an oily, yellow pigment that appears to prevent gut muscles from contracting and cramping.

What else turmeric can do: relieve arthritis, morning stiffness and minor sprains. Turmeric reduces levels of an inflammatory, hormone-like substance known as *PGE2*. In lab studies, researchers also are finding that turmeric helps prevent colorectal and skin cancers, but its cancer-fighting mechanism has not yet been identified.

In addition, turmeric is being studied for its possible role in decreasing risk for Alzheimer's disease. Test tube and animal studies suggest that turmeric interferes with the formation of amyloid plaque, a hallmark of this neurodegenerative disease.

Recommended: Consume turmeric powder regularly by adding it to food, such as Asian dishes.

Caution: Because turmeric can cause gallbladder contractions, people with gallbladder problems should avoid the herb.

Turmeric: The Spice That May Prevent Alzheimer's

Mark A. Stengler, NMD, naturopathic medical doctor in private practice, Encinitas, California...adjunct associate clinical professor at the National College of Natural Medicine, Portland, Oregon...author of many books, including *The Natural Physician's Healing Therapies* and coauthor of *Prescription for Natural Cures* (both from Bottom Line Books)...and author of the *Bottom Line/Natural Healing* newsletter.

In India, the smell of turmeric, the bright yellow spice used in curries, fills almost every restaurant and home. Indians eat turmeric because they like it, but rapidly growing evidence indicates that the spice is giving them much more than flavor.

Thousands of years ago, Ayurvedic and traditional Chinese medicine recognized turmeric as a healing agent for everything from flatulence to liver disease. Now modern research demonstrates that properties in this zesty spice may be useful for lowering rates of breast, prostate, lung and colon cancers, and also for treating breast cancer, inflammatory bowel disease, Crohn's disease and possibly cystic fibrosis.

But even newer and especially exciting research concerns the relationship between turmeric and Alzheimer's disease. Nearly 10 years ago, researchers in India became curious about the influence turmeric might have on rates of Alzheimer's. They looked to see how many people over age 65 in a town in India had signs of the disease, versus a similar group of people in a similar-sized Pennsylvania town, where most people eat little—or no—turmeric.

What they found: In India, just 4.7 per 1,000 person-years (a common measure of incidence rate) showed signs of Alzheimer's, compared with a rate of 17.5 per 1,000 person-years in Pennsylvania. In fact, India has among the lowest rates of Alzheimer's disease in the world. Another study, from the National University of Singapore, involved 1,010 people over age 60. Those who reported that they ate curry "often or very often" or even "occasionally" scored higher on mental performance tests than those who rarely or never consumed it.

WHAT IS TURMERIC?

Turmeric is a powder made from the root of the plant *Curcuma longa*, which grows in southern Asia. The part of the plant that is responsible for healing is the yellow pigment, called *curcumin*.

When it comes to health-giving properties, curcumin gives twice. It is a potent anti-inflammatory agent, without the potential side effects of anti-inflammatory drugs. These include damage to the lining of the stomach and intestines and a greater risk for kidney and liver problems, heart attack and stroke. Next, curcumin is a powerful antioxidant—it tracks down and reduces free radicals, molecules that otherwise would cause damage in the body. Both of these properties are important when it comes to preventing or slowing the progression of Alzheimer's disease.

In healthy people, immune cells attack and destroy amyloid-beta plaques—a buildup of proteins between neurons in the brain. But in people with Alzheimer's, this immune response is less efficient and allows plaques to form. Plaque triggers inflammation and free radicals, both of which cause cell damage in the brain. Curcumin slows this harmful process in a number of ways—it forms a powerful bond with the amyloid protein that prevents the protein from clumping...it may break down plaques as well, preliminary research demonstrates...and finally, as I noted before, curcumin reduces the oxidative damage and brain inflammation that are linked to Alzheimer's disease.

CHOLESTEROL BLASTER

There is yet more good news about curcumin's power to prevent and even fight Alzheimer's disease. Elevated cholesterol is thought to be involved in the development of Alzheimer's—and studies demonstrate that curcumin reduces cholesterol. In one study, healthy volunteers took 500 milligrams (mg) of curcumin supplements every day for one week.

Result: Reduced levels of total cholesterol and also *lipid peroxides* (markers of free radical damage to fats).

SPICE UP YOUR DIET

In the meantime, I encourage all my patients, especially those over age 50, to consume one or two teaspoons a day of turmeric. There are many ways to incorporate this spice into your regular diet. You can sprinkle it into egg salad or over vegetables while sautéing...add it to soups or broths...put it on fish or meat...and use it to flavor rice or a creamy vegetable dip. And of course, turmeric adds zing to curries. If you want to make the most healthful curry dishes, it is important to purchase turmeric as a separate spice—lab tests show that many curry powders in this country contain almost no turmeric.

Good brand: Indus Organics, Inc. (*www.greatorganicspices.com*, $5.99 for six ounces).

Those who don't love turmeric—or those who want to get even more of its protective effects—can take curcumin in supplement form. I prescribe 2,000 mg a day for people who have a strong family history of Alzheimer's disease or who show signs of dementia.

Good brands: New Chapter Turmericforce (800-543-7279, *www.newchapter.com*) and Life Extension Super Curcumin with Bioperine (800-544-4440, *www.lef.org*).

Anyone taking blood-thinning drugs should discuss using turmeric or curcumin supplements with a doctor, because curcumin is a natural blood thinner. Turmeric also can cause gallbladder contractions, so those with a history of gallstones or gallbladder problems also should consult a doctor. There is no risk in mixing curcumin with pharmaceutical drugs for Alzheimer's disease.

Gingerroot—Not Just For Cookies

Mark A. Stengler, NMD, naturopathic medical doctor in private practice, Encinitas, California...adjunct associate clinical professor at the National College of Natural Medicine, Portland, Oregon...author of many books, including *The Natural Physician's Healing Therapies* and coauthor of *Prescription for Natural Cures* (both from Bottom Line Books)...and author of the *Bottom Line/Natural Healing* newsletter.

For centuries, ginger (*Zingiber officinale*) has been widely valued as a medicinal herb. It is one of the most widely prescribed herbs by practitioners of Ayurvedic and Chinese traditional medicines. The botanical name for ginger is *zingiber*, which, in Sanskrit, means "shaped like a horn." Technically speaking, the root is actually a rhizome, a stem that runs underneath the surface of the ground.

It's most commonly used to treat digestive disorders and arthritis in all the healing traditions. It is known as a warming herb, especially suited to people with "cold constitutions," and it's said to enhance circulation. Chinese herbalists use fresh ginger to "warm the lung and stomach."

Ginger is prescribed in Chinese medicine for the common cold, flu, coughs, vomiting, nausea and general digestive upset and bleeding. It also reduces the toxicity of other herbs, so it's essentially an antidote to plants that might have side effects. Also, ginger can help protect an intestinal tract that has been ravaged by tainted or toxic food.

To practitioners of traditional Chinese medicine, every form of gingerroot has certain distinct properties. Fresh ginger has a warming effect on the exterior of the body, while the dried ginger is apt to be recommended for warming the middle of the body.

One of the more intriguing Chinese medicine cures is quick-fried ginger, which is made by frying ginger until the surface is slightly blackened. Practitioners say this is the type that's effective for stopping bleeding and treating conditions that affect the lower abdomen.

Today, ginger is used by herbalists and physicians to treat colds, arthritis, digestive conditions, respiratory-tract infections, headaches, motion sickness and cardiovascular disease.

As with many herbs, ginger has many different active constituents. Dried gingerroot contains between 1% and 4% volatile oils, which account for the strong taste and aroma. (The volatile oils include *bisabolene*, *zingiberene* and *zingiberol*.) Two of the pungent principles—*gingerol* and *shogaol*—are believed to be responsible for a lot of the medicinal effects.

Ginger also contains proteolytic enzymes that help to digest proteins and reduce inflammation. Many commercial products are standardized to the constituent gingerol.

DIGESTIVE POWER

Ginger has the unique ability to improve many organs that are involved with digestion. Known as an "aromatic bitter," it tonifies the intestinal muscles and stimulates the digestive organs. It also stimulates secretion of bile from the liver and gallbladder, which helps digest fats. Ginger is also a well-known *carminative*, meaning that it can reduce gas and bloating.

ANTI-INFLAMMATORY

Ginger acts as a natural anti-inflammatory by inhibiting the release of prostaglandins and other chemicals in the body that promote inflammation and pain. Unlike nonsteroidal medications such as aspirin, it does not have the potential to damage the stomach, liver and kidneys. For centuries, people used ginger as an anti-inflammatory without knowing how or why it worked. Modern tests have now proven the herb's anti-inflammatory powers.

CIRCULATION AND CARDIOVASCULAR HEALTH

Ginger promotes cardiovascular health by making platelets (cells responsible for blood clots) less likely to clump together. This preventive action allows the blood to keep flowing smoothly and helps prevent hardening of the arteries.

Studies have shown that this protective effect is achieved by inhibiting the formation of *thromboxanes*, substances that promote blood clotting. Other substances in ginger promote the synthesis of *prostacyclin*, a component that helps prevent platelets from "aggregating" or clumping together.

Animal studies have also shown that ginger improves the pumping ability of the heart.

Dosage: Fresh gingerroot can be made into tea. It's also sold in capsules, tablets, and tinctures. I have found all these forms to work with patients and myself.

The tea is relaxing and works well for digestive upset, as do the capsule and tincture forms. For the treatment of inflammatory conditions, I recommend a standardized capsule to get high levels of the active constituents that reduce inflammation.

The typical capsule dosage is 500 milligrams (mg) two to four times daily. If you're taking the tincture, I recommend 20 to 30 drops two to three times daily.

What are the side effects? Side effects are rare with ginger, though some people (my wife among them!) report heartburn after taking it. In the short term, pregnant women can take ginger for nausea and vomiting related to morning sickness. One to two grams (g) appear to be safe and effective.

Ginger stimulates bile production, so some herbal experts recommend that you should avoid this herb if you have gallstones.

Although I have seen no human studies on drug interactions and ginger, it theoretically may cause a problem with blood-thinning medications such as *warfarin* (Coumadin). So check with your physician before using high doses of ginger if you are on a blood-thinning medication.

One last piece of advice you may not find in many books is that gingerroot by itself may aggravate those who are very warm-blooded. If you are the type of person who gets warm and sweats easily, then long-term use of ginger is not recommended just because it can cause discomfort by making you even warmer.

Healing Spices: Surprising New Discoveries

David Winston, RH, a Washington, New Jersey–based registered herbalist and professional member of the American Herbalist Guild. He is author of several books, including *Adaptogens: Herbs for Strength, Stamina and Stress Relief* (Healing Arts).

Researchers have now identified new health benefits for several popular spices. You may recognize the names of these spices, but the latest studies suggest uses that are not widely known. *Intriguing research...*

CAYENNE PEPPER

• **Cholesterol.** Artery-clogging fatty build-ups are created or worsened when cholesterol oxidizes, a biochemical process similar to metal rusting. Cayenne pepper (also known as chili pepper) contains a plaque-fighting antioxidant (*capsaicin*), which is also available in supplement form.

Recent research: When researchers asked 27 people to eat a diet that included cayenne-spiced chili or the same diet with no chili for one month, the spicy-chili group had much lower harmful cholesterol than those who did not eat chili. In addition to protecting cholesterol from oxidation, cayenne pepper also stimulates digestion and improves circulation—an important benefit for people with chronically cold hands and feet.

Recommendation: Use a cayenne-based hot sauce, to taste. Add it to a variety of foods, including chicken dishes and sandwiches.

Caution: In some people, cayenne causes digestive problems. If you experience stomach upset or anal irritation, use a milder hot sauce, cut back the amount or stop using it.

SAGE

• **Alzheimer's disease.** Herbalists and many doctors report that sage may help patients with mild to moderate Alzheimer's disease.

Newest research: Neurons of lab animals exposed to *amyloid-beta* (the main constituent of harmful plaques in Alzheimer's) and sage leaves or *rosmarinic acid* (an active ingredient in sage) were less damaged than when the cells were exposed to amyloid-beta alone. However, you cannot achieve this potential health benefit from the amount of sage used in cooking.

My recommendation: Drink sage tea.

What to do: Pour eight ounces of boiling water over a tea strainer or tea ball that contains one-half teaspoon of ground sage. Let sit for 15 to 20 minutes. Drink four ounces twice a day. (Refrigerate any unused portion and gently reheat before drinking.)

Alternative: Use sage tea bags. Or add 20 to 30 drops of sage tincture to one ounce of water—drink this amount three times daily.

ROSEMARY

• **Cancer.** Laboratory studies of human cells show that rosemary may help prevent certain types of cancer.

Recent research: The rate at which human leukemia and breast cancer cells multiplied in a laboratory study was reduced when researchers exposed the cells to rosemary extract. More research is needed to confirm these benefits in human study subjects, but rosemary extract is safe to use in the meantime. Cooking with rosemary does not provide this potential health benefit.

Recommendation: Drink rosemary tea.

What to do: Pour 12 ounces of boiling water over a tea strainer or tea ball that contains one-half teaspoon of rosemary. Let sit for 15 to 20 minutes. Drink four ounces, three times a day. (Refrigerate unused tea.)

Alternative: Use rosemary tea bags. Or add 40 to 60 drops of rosemary tincture to one ounce of water—drink this amount three times daily.

HOW TO USE SPICES

The active ingredients in spices can eventually deteriorate after processing. For example, the levels of antioxidants, known as carotenoids, in paprika drop by 75% after three months of storage.

Recommendation: Buy no more than a one-year supply of any spice you plan to use—and replace it annually. Keep your spices away from light, moisture and heat—for example, not near the oven. Consider buying whole rather than powdered spices, and grind them right before using, with a mortar and pestle or spice grinder. To tell whether a spice is rich in health-promoting compounds, smell and/or taste it—the richer the odor and flavor, the better the spice.

---

7 Must-Have Healing Herbs

Kathy Abascal, RH, a registered herbalist who practices in Vashon, Washington. A member of the American Herbalists Guild, she is coauthor of *Clinical Botanical Medicine* (Mary Ann Liebert).

Until recently, if you peeked inside the medicine cabinet of a typical American household, you were likely to find such items as aspirin for headaches...an anti-inflammatory ointment for sore muscles and joints...an antihistamine for colds—and perhaps even a prescription sedative for sleep problems and/or an antidepressant.

Latest development: With the recent economic downturn and rising drug costs, many Americans are turning to medicinal alternatives. In 2009, nationwide sales of herbal supplements totaled $5 billion, up nearly 5% from the previous year. Perhaps due to the recession, Americans now appear to be trying many of the same herb-based products that have been used for generations in other parts of the world as the front-line treatments for many common conditions.

How herbs can help you: Compared with many medications widely used in the US, herbal therapies tend to have fewer side effects, are generally just as effective—if not more so—and are often less expensive.*

Seven of the most useful herbs to have on hand in your home...

ECHINACEA FOR COLDS

One study reported that echinacea is not effective for the common cold. Later research found that it does help. Does it or doesn't it?

Echinacea stimulates both white blood cells (which attack viruses) and natural killer cells (which destroy virus-infected cells). Most scientific studies of echinacea involve dosing patients every four to six hours. That's not enough.

How to use: Add about one teaspoon of echinacea tincture to one-half cup of water. Drink it once every waking hour at the first signs of a cold until symptoms subside.

Helpful: Add to the mixture one-half teaspoon of elderberry tincture—which also helps boost immunity—for additional antiviral effects.

EUCALYPTUS FOR CONGESTION

Used as an essential oil, eucalyptus penetrates the mucous membranes and promotes drainage—helpful for relieving symptoms caused by the common cold and/or sinusitis (inflammation of the sinuses). The oil also has antimicrobial properties that can inhibit viruses and bacteria.

How to use: At the first signs of a cold or sinusitis, put five to 10 drops of eucalyptus essential oil in a large bowl. Add one to two cups of steaming hot water. (The dose is correct if you can smell the eucalyptus.) Put a towel over your head, and lean over the bowl (with your eyes closed) and breathe in the steam for about 10 minutes. Repeat as needed, using fresh eucalyptus oil each time.

Caution: Keep your head far enough from the steaming water to avoid burning yourself.

TURMERIC FOR JOINT PAIN

Studies show that this extremely potent anti-inflammatory herb is about as effective as nonsteroidal anti-inflammatory drugs—such as aspirin and *ibuprofen* (Advil)—for easing joint pain. Unlike these and similar drugs, turmeric

*If you have a chronic condition and/or take prescription medication, consult your doctor before taking herbs.

(taken at the doses recommended below) rarely causes stomach upset or other side effects.

How to use: Take 400 milligrams (mg) to 500 mg, three times daily. For additional benefits, use powdered turmeric when cooking. As little as one-quarter teaspoon per recipe will have anti-inflammatory effects over time.

Important: When cooking, use turmeric and black pepper. This greatly increases absorption of turmeric into the bloodstream.

Also helpful: Look for a turmeric supplement formula that includes black pepper.

VALERIAN FOR INSOMNIA

Compounds in valerian act on brain receptors to induce drowsiness and relaxation.

How to use: Take one-half teaspoon of valerian tincture, diluted in water according to the instructions on the label, one hour before bedtime and one-half teaspoon at bedtime, as needed. In small doses—about one-quarter to one-half of the insomnia dose—valerian also can help reduce mild anxiety. Most people avoid valerian tea due to its unpleasant odor.

WHITE WILLOW BARK FOR HEADACHES

It contains *salicin*, a chemical that's converted in the body into salicylic acid, an aspirin-like substance. Some studies indicate that white willow bark works as well as aspirin (minus the side effects, such as gastrointestinal upset) for headaches and other types of pain, such as osteoarthritis pain and low-back pain.

How to use: Take 200 mg, twice daily with food for headache and other types of pain (described above).

Caution: If you take a blood thinner, such as *warfarin* (Coumadin), consult your physician before using white willow bark, which also has blood-thinning effects.

ST. JOHN'S WORT TO LIFT YOUR MOOD

It's thought to inhibit the activity of enzymes that break down *serotonin*, a neurotransmitter that plays a key role in regulating mood.

Studies have shown that St. John's wort is as effective for mild to moderate depression as some prescription antidepressants.

St. John's wort also is one of the most effective herbs for treating seasonal affective disorder (SAD), a form of depression that tends to occur in winter.

Caution: Consult your doctor before trying St. John's wort if you take a prescription antidepressant or other medication—or drink alcohol.

How to use: The recommended dose is usually 300 mg, three times daily (standardized to 0.3% *hypericin*). Consult your doctor for advice on treatment duration.

Helpful: If you suffer from SAD, take 1,000 international units (IU) to 2,000 IU of vitamin D along with St. John's wort. A lack of sun and low levels of vitamin D (which is also associated with infrequent sun exposure) can cause depression.

ALOE VERA FOR BURNS

Like an antibiotic cream, the gel from aloe leaves has antimicrobial properties. It soothes painful burns.

How to use: Keep an aloe plant in your home. For minor burns, slice open an aloe leaf and squeeze the gel over the affected area. Store-bought aloe gel also is effective.

Helpful: Keep several aloe leaves in the freezer. The cold gel from the frozen leaves will act as a mild anesthetic.

Echinacea—the Best-Selling Immune Booster

Mark A. Stengler, NMD, naturopathic medical doctor in private practice, Encinitas, California...adjunct associate clinical professor at the National College of Natural Medicine, Portland, Oregon...author of many books, including *The Natural Physician's Healing Therapies* and coauthor of *Prescription for Natural Cures* (both from Bottom Line Books)...and author of the *Bottom Line/Natural Healing* newsletter.

It's not unusual to get calls at my office from patients wondering what to do about the cold or flu that just hit them.

My first thought is: What natural supplements can they get quickly, right off the shelf?

Well, just about anyone can find echinacea (pronounced eck-in-ay'-sha) at a nearby store.

It's one of the five top-selling herbs in North America. In fact, it's a worldwide best-seller, as herbalists and doctors in Europe have been prescribing echinacea for decades. Carrying the popular name of purple coneflower (so-called because of its purple, daisy-like petals), echinacea is renowned as an herb that enhances the immune system. It's commonly used to treat a number of conditions from flu and the common cold to a range of other infectious diseases.

INFECTION FIGHTER TO THE RESCUE

Echinacea as a healing remedy was introduced to Europe during the 1930s. Since then the preponderance of scientific research on echinacea has been done in Western Europe, especially Germany, where the government plays an active role in funding research on natural medicine. But Canadian and American researchers have recently made similar strides in echinacea research, with clinical studies and biochemical analysis of the healing herb.

Over 400 studies to date have looked at the pharmacology and clinical uses of echinacea. Not all studies have shown efficacy of the herb, but most of the research indicates that echinacea helps reinforce the immune system.

Echinacea is consistently one of the best-selling herbs in North America and Europe. Over 10 million units are sold annually in Germany alone.

Though there are nine species of echinacea, *Echinacea purpurea* and *Echinacea angustifolia* are the two most often used commercially. Most clinical studies are done with these species, especially purpurea.

AROUSING IMMUNE CELLS

Echinacea doesn't work like the pharmaceutical antibiotics that "kill" microbes like bacteria. Instead, echinacea arouses the immune cells that patrol and defend the body against these invaders. It increases the number and activity of disease-fighting white blood cells, and it activates antiviral chemicals such as *interferon*. Echinacea can even activate the immune cells that fight tumors. In addition, research has shown that the chemicals in echinacea have the power to inhibit an enzyme released by bacteria, called *hyaluronidase*. Bacteria normally produce this enzyme to penetrate into human tissue. Echinacea prevents this from happening.

Researchers in a German study found clear evidence that echinacea helps to promote good immune cells, called *phagocytes*. One group of people were given 30 drops of echinacea three times daily for five days, while people in the control group were given a placebo. The level of phagocytes was measured at the beginning and throughout the study. At day three, the phagocyte activity of those taking echinacea increased by 40 percent. By the fifth day, phagocyte activity had increased 120 percent. When people stopped taking echinacea, immune-cell activity dropped off sharply. After three days, there was no difference in immune-cell activity between the group taking echinacea and the control group.

Leading researchers now feel that echinacea may be more of an immune-modulating herb, meaning it has a balancing effect on the immune system. As research continues, this may mean that echinacea may be more valuable than just boosting immune function.

VIRUS SLAYERS

While there are a host of modern antibiotics for killing bacteria, modern medicine has a limited arsenal of weapons to defeat viral infections. This presents a problem for the many doctors who rely on conventional pharmaceuticals in their medical practice. Over 65 million people in the U.S. each year "catch" the common cold, while another 108 million get the flu—and these are just two of the infectious diseases caused by viruses. Others include genital herpes, which affects an estimated 45 million people, as well as hepatitis C, which afflicts 170 million people in the world. Even a simple viral infection like a viral sore throat poses a challenge for any doctor who relies exclusively on antibiotics and other conventional prescription medications.

Echinacea, like other immune-enhancing herbs, has a direct antiviral effect. Even better, it seems to summon all the resources of the immune system to help destroy invading viruses.

It also works well in combination with other antiviral plants and herbs. I like to prescribe echinacea in a formula called the "virus cocktail," which is comprised of echinacea, lomatium, astragalus, reishi and licorice root. The synergistic blend of these herbs tends to be more effective than any one herb by itself.

BACTERIA AND FUNGUS

Since echinacea enhances the action of your immune cells, it is also effective against bacterial, fungal and yeast infections. This is especially helpful if you're fighting a bacterial infection, because many bacteria are now resistant to antibiotics (because they're overprescribed by doctors for things like viral infections). If needed, there is no problem using echinacea in combination with antibiotics. As a matter of fact, I find when people are on antibiotics for a bacterial infection and use echinacea simultaneously, they recover more quickly.

Dosage: Echinacea is generally available as a tincture, capsule, tablet or cream in the US. It's also possible to take it in the form of an injection, though this method is mainly used in Germany.

Glycerine (alcohol-free) tinctures are available. These are good for kids, who especially enjoy the berry-flavored varieties.

- **Tincture.** I recommend 20 to 60 drops of the tincture every two to three hours for acute infections or twice daily for long-term use.

- **Capsule.** I recommend 500 to 1,000 milligrams every two to three hours for acute infections or twice daily for long-term use.

Note: High-potency, quality echinacea products are standardized to contain active ingredients such as *alkylamides*, *cichoric acid* and *polysaccharides*.

Some controversy surrounds the length of time one can use echinacea. Many authors state that echinacea should not be used on a long-term basis. However, there are no studies showing that long-term use is harmful or that echinacea loses its effectiveness.

I generally recommend patients use echinacea for acute infections until they are completely over the illness. For those who are very susceptible to infections, especially during the winter, and do not want to change their lifestyle, echinacea can be used on a long-term basis (although it is not so effective as improving diet, reducing stress and exercising). Long-term use of echinacea throughout the winter season is common in European countries.

Ginkgo Biloba—a Power Plant

Mark A. Stengler, NMD, naturopathic medical doctor in private practice, Encinitas, California...adjunct associate clinical professor at the National College of Natural Medicine, Portland, Oregon...author of many books, including *The Natural Physician's Healing Therapies* and coauthor of *Prescription for Natural Cures* (both from Bottom Line Books)...and author of the *Bottom Line/ Natural Healing* newsletter.

Ginkgo ranks among the top five herbs that I prescribe to patients on a daily basis. Millions of people around the world use ginkgo every day. In countries such as Germany and France, where doctors are accustomed to writing herbal prescriptions, ginkgo is among the most commonly prescribed medicines. European doctors use it to treat a wide range of conditions—from memory impairment, dizziness and ringing in the ears (tinnitus) to headaches and depression. There are even more uses—such as a blood mover for improved circulation.

Fossil records show that the ginkgo is the world's oldest living species of tree. It's very hardy, able to thrive in extreme heat and cold, and to withstand the sinus-hammering pollution of downtown Los Angeles or New York. It's also almost pest-proof—there doesn't seem to be an insect that can do serious damage to this hardy tree.

The leaves, the source of ginkgo medicinals, are fan-shaped and bilobed (divided into two sections), resembling the maidenhair fern. The resemblance is so close, it's sometimes called the "maidenhair tree."

TURNING OVER AN OLD LEAF

Researchers in the 1950s, having heard of the medicinal powers of ginkgo (tree) leaves, began mashing and distilling the components in search of the so-called active ingredients—

that is, the chemical compounds that seemed to have potential healing power. What are believed to be the key medicinal ingredients have now been identified.

The two groups of active components include *flavone glycosides* and *terpene lactones*. Quality ginkgo products are "standardized" to 24% flavone glycosides and 6% terpene lactones—which is a virtual guarantee that the products contain at least these proportions of those particular ingredients. Such products have the same proportion of these ingredients as the extract that's used in clinical studies.

POTENT CELL PROTECTOR

Flavone glycosides are types of bioflavonoids, the plant-based compounds that are found in oranges and other fruits and vegetables. With bioflavonoids, ginkgo has been blessed with the potent powers of an antioxidant. That means if you take ginkgo, you're less likely to suffer the cellular damage caused by free radicals—unstable molecules that are a result of metabolic activities in the body and environmental pollution.

Many researchers believe that ginkgo produces more antioxidant activity than many of the better-known vitamin antioxidants such as C, E and beta carotene. Several studies have demonstrated that ginkgo exerts antioxidant activity in the brain, eyes and cardiovascular system. This could easily explain why ginkgo seems to be effective in the prevention and treatment of diseases that affect those parts of the body—including Alzheimer's disease, strokes, cataracts, macular degeneration and diabetic retinopathy.

Ginkgo bioflavonoids also protect blood vessels by strengthening and reducing inflammation of their elastic walls. So that's an additional benefit of this herb—significant in helping to relieve varicose veins and reverse the effects of cardiovascular disease.

KEEPING UP CIRCULATION

In addition to the bioflavonoids, ginkgo has another component, unique to this plant. A family of terpene lactones, specifically called *ginkgolides* and *bilobalides*, give ginkgo an extraordinary ability to increase circulation to the brain and extremities. The substances cause the blood vessel walls to relax and dilate, which permits increased blood flow. They also have what's called a "tonifying effect" on the venous system, allowing for the more efficient return of blood to the heart.

Ginkgo also has a natural blood-thinning effect. It helps to prevent blood platelets from sticking together—and platelets are the cells that form blood clots.

The way ginkgo improves circulation is particularly impressive. In one study measuring blood flow through capillaries in healthy adults, researchers found a 57 percent increase in blood flow in those taking ginkgo. As we age, we're more likely to have blockages in the blood flow that reaches the brain and other parts of the bodies. These problems are directly attributable to plaque buildup in the arteries. Ginkgo acts as sort of a bypass mechanism, helping the blood make its way through partially clogged arteries.

NERVE RENEWAL

The ginkgolides also help protect nerve cells from being damaged. This is important for people who are recovering from a stroke. In addition, some ongoing research will probably show whether ginkgo has the benefits that it's reputed to possess for people who are recovering from brain trauma. What's certain is that nerve cells need the kind of protection that ginkgo provides—particularly people (such as those with diabetes) who have problems with neuropathy (nerve disorder).

Dosage: As a standard dosage, I recommend a ginkgo extract standardized to 24% flavone glycosides and 6% terpene lactones. Dosages used in studies range from 120 milligrams (mg) to 360 mg daily. Most of my patients take 60 mg two to four times daily, for a daily total of 120 to 240 mg. The vast majority report beneficial results.

For severe cases, like early-stage Alzheimer's disease, I recommend that people take 240 to 360 mg daily.

If you start to take ginkgo for a particular condition or for general health, I suggest you continue taking it for at least eight weeks to assess its therapeutic effect. Most of my patients who take it to improve their memory or help their circulation notice the beginnings of improvements within about a month.

Ginkgo supplements are available in capsule, tablet and tincture form.

What are the side effects? Doctors, researchers and practitioners have noted very few adverse effects among people who take ginkgo. A small number—less than 1 percent of those who take it—have reported mild digestive upset.

Other rare side effects mentioned in the literature include headaches and dizziness. I've had very few patients who complained of these problems, and in those few cases, the side effects disappeared when I lowered the dosage.

One warning, however. If you're taking a blood-thinning medication such as *warfarin* (Coumadin) or aspirin, be sure to notify your doctor. These medications, like ginkgo, have a blood-thinning effect—and the cumulative doses might be more than you need. Your doctor can monitor how well your blood is clotting through regular blood work, by taking blood samples and testing them in the lab.

My recommendations for...

- **Alzheimer's disease.**

Dosage: 240–360 mg.

- **Circulatory diseases** (as well as other conditions that involve poor circulation).

Dosage: 120–160 mg.

- **Depression.**

Dosage: 240 mg.

- **High blood pressure.**

Dosage: 120–180 mg daily.

- **Impotence.**

Dosage: 180–240 mg.

ALSO GOOD FOR

- **Premenstrual syndrome (PMS).**
- **Radiation effects.**
- **Ringing in the ears (tinnitus).**
- **Stroke.**
- **Vision problems** (macular degeneration, diabetic retinopathy, and cataracts).

If You Take Herbs...Read This *Before* You Have Surgery

David J. Rowe, MD, assistant professor in the department of plastic surgery at University Hospitals Case Medical Center in Cleveland.

Every patient is asked before surgery, "What medications do you take?" Yet 40% to 70% of patients do not report their use of herbal supplements—typically because they don't think of supplements as medication.

The concern: Though many herbs generally are safe, when you are undergoing or recovering from surgery—even a minor procedure—certain herbs can lead to potentially serious side effects, such as...

BLEEDING PROBLEMS

Some herbs thin the blood, possibly complicating surgery and delaying healing. *These include...*

- **Dong quai,** commonly used for menstrual cramps and menopausal symptoms.
- **Feverfew,** for arthritis and headache.
- **Garlic,** which is taken to stimulate the immune system.
- **Ginkgo biloba,** used for eye disorders, cognitive problems and vertigo.
- **Ginseng,** used for stress.

CARDIOVASCULAR SIDE EFFECTS

Postoperative hypertension, heart palpitations or other serious heart problems may develop if you are taking...

- **Feverfew,** for arthritis and headache.
- **Garlic,** for immune-strengthening.

DRUG INTERACTIONS

The actions and side effects of drugs commonly given before, during or after surgery—such as *lidocaine* (an anesthetic) and *midazolam* (a sedative)—may be intensified by...

- **Echinacea,** for cold and flu.
- **Goldenseal,** taken to relieve digestive and respiratory problems.

PHOTOSENSITIVITY

If you have laser surgery, you may develop a severe light-sensitivity rash if you are taking...

- **Dong quai,** for menstrual and menopausal symptoms.
- **St. John's wort,** for anxiety.
- **Reaction to anesthesia.**
- **Herbs that prolong sedation...**
  - Kava, a sedative.
  - St. John's wort, for anxiety, depression.
  - Valerian, for insomnia.

Self-defense: Follow these steps...

- **A month before any scheduled surgery,** give your doctor a list of every supplement and medication that you take.
- **Even if your doctor is not concerned,** it is safest to discontinue all supplements at least two weeks before surgery.
- **On the day of your operation,** remind your surgeon about any recent supplement use. Also show your list to the anesthesiologist.
- **Carry a personal health record that lists all supplements and drugs you take**—so that if you need emergency surgery, doctors can take precautions.
- **After surgery,** wait until your doctor declares you sufficiently healed before you resume supplementing.

EXCEPTIONS

Though clinical research is limited, anecdotal evidence suggests that recovery may be hastened by...

- **Arnica,** used for pain and inflammation.
- **Bromelain,** an enzyme with analgesic and anti-inflammatory properties.

With your doctor's okay, consider taking arnica and/or bromelain (following dosage instructions on labels) starting the day after surgery.

SPECIAL REPORT #4

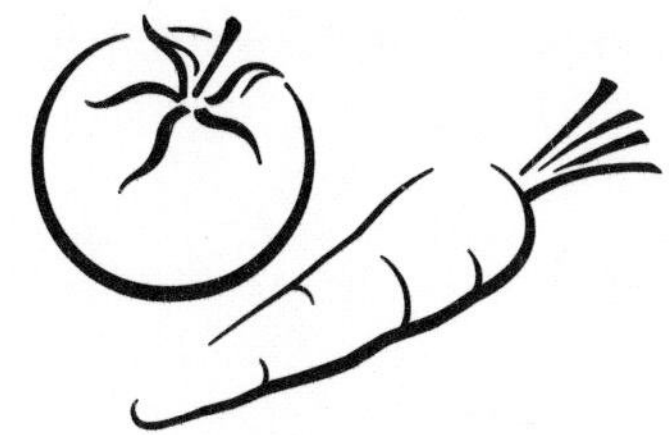

Best-Ever Healing Food Combinations

Best-Ever Healing Food Combinations

Supercharge Your Meals

Until recently, most nutrition research has focused on the health benefits of individual nutrients. For example, it's well-established that vitamin A is good for the eyes...calcium builds stronger bones...and zinc boosts immunity.

Now there is strong scientific evidence that nutrition is much more complex than that. When certain foods are combined, their nutritional value is much greater than when the foods are eaten individually.

That's why dietitians recommend eating a varied diet with plenty of fruits, vegetables, whole grains and low-fat proteins—the greater the variety, the better your chances of maximizing the health benefits of your food.

Latest development: Scientists are beginning to understand exactly which specific food combinations are the most effective in helping the body fight common ailments.

For example...

TO FIGHT ARTHRITIS

- **Combine carotenes and spices.** Carotenes are a group of powerful antioxidants that attack toxic, cell-damaging molecules known as free radicals.

In addition to the familiar beta-carotene, there are other carotenes, including *beta-cryptoxanthin*, which has been shown to fight rheumatoid arthritis and osteoarthritis.

Good sources of both beta-carotene and beta-cryptoxanthin: Winter squash (especially butternut), pumpkin, red bell peppers and carrots...apricots and watermelon.

The spices turmeric (with its antioxidant oil curcumin) and ginger contain phytochemicals that help suppress inflammatory reactions that can lead to arthritis. Turmeric is the bright yellow, dried spice found in curry powder. Ginger

Joy Bauer, RD, CDN, author of several nutrition books, including *Joy's LIFE Diet: 4 Steps to Thin Forever* (Collins Living) and *Joy Bauer's Food Cures* (Rodale). Bauer is the nutrition expert for the Today show and has a private practice with offices in New York City and Westchester County, New York. *www.joybauer.com.*

is available in powdered form as a spice and also as a fresh root.

My favorite arthritis-fighting combos: Curried butternut squash soup…pumpkin and ginger muffins…Asian ginger stir-fry with red bell peppers…and curried carrots.

TO FIGHT HEART PROBLEMS

•Combine lycopene and monounsaturated fats. Lycopene is a fat-soluble antioxidant that has been shown to reduce the risk for heart disease, perhaps by stopping the process that leads to atherosclerosis (fatty buildup in the arteries).

Good sources of lycopene: Tomatoes, red and pink grapefruit, watermelon and guava.

Helpful: Eat cooked tomatoes—they contain three to four times more lycopene than raw tomatoes.

Monounsaturated fats are believed to protect against heart disease and have a number of cardiovascular benefits. These healthful fats help the body absorb all fat-soluble nutrients, including lycopene.

Good sources of monounsaturated fats: Olive oil and canola oil…avocado…almonds, walnuts, peanuts and cashews.

My favorite heart-healthy combos: Roasted tomatoes with a touch of olive oil…any meal made with homemade or store-bought tomato sauce that contains olive oil…a salad of grapefruit and avocado…and turkey, avocado and tomato sandwiches.

TO FIGHT MEMORY LOSS

•Combine folic acid and anthocyanins. One of the B vitamins, folic acid (also known as folate) helps lower blood levels of the amino acid *homocysteine*—a process that research suggests may promote blood flow to the brain. Folic acid also enhances communication between neurotransmitters, which are chemicals in the brain.

Good sources of folic acid: Fortified whole-grain breakfast cereals and oatmeal…green, leafy vegetables, bok choy and broccoli…oranges (or orange juice) and berries (such as strawberries and blackberries).

Anthocyanins are antioxidant phytochemicals that have been shown to not only help prevent memory loss but also improve failing memory.

Good sources of anthocyanins: Berries (especially blueberries—their antioxidant *flavonols* help protect against brain degeneration), red or black grapes…red or purple cabbage, beets, red onions and eggplant.

My favorite memory-enhancing combos: Folic acid–fortified breakfast cereal with berries…coleslaw with red cabbage and bok choy…chicken-vegetable stir-fry with red onions and broccoli…and fruit salad with oranges and blueberries.

TO FIGHT FATIGUE

•Combine iron and vitamin C. Iron helps red blood cells carry oxygen throughout the body. Without enough iron, your cells can become starved for oxygen. This can lead to anemia, which causes listlessness, headache, irritability and general lack of energy.

Good sources of iron: Lean beef, turkey, chicken, lamb and pork…clams, oysters and shrimp…soybeans, chickpeas and lentils…spinach, asparagus and green, leafy vegetables.

Vitamin C is a powerful antioxidant, but most people don't realize that it can help fight fatigue by enhancing the body's ability to absorb iron. By adding a food that contains significant amounts of vitamin C to a meal with an iron-rich food, your body will absorb up to three times more iron.

This is especially important for vegetarians, premenopausal women (who lose iron through menstruation) and people with a genetic predisposition to anemia (determined through blood tests).

Caution: People with *hemochromatosis*, a dangerous disorder that causes iron to build up in the blood, should not combine foods high in iron and vitamin C.

Good sources of vitamin C: Bell and hot chili peppers, broccoli and kale…tomatoes, mangoes, oranges (or orange juice), strawberries and pineapple.

My favorite fatigue-fighting combos: Spinach salad with mandarin oranges…bean chili (such as kidney, pinto or black bean) with crushed tomatoes…steak with sautéed broccoli…and chicken cacciatore with tomatoes and peppers.

TO FIGHT MOOD SWINGS

•**Combine soluble fiber and protein.** Mood swings often are caused by fluctuations in blood sugar (glucose).

Low-quality carbohydrates, such as white rice, white bread, cakes and soft drinks, cause blood sugar spikes that usually lead to a sluggish, depressed feeling about one hour after consumption of such foods.

High-quality carbohydrates, such as vegetables, fruits and whole grains, contain soluble fiber that causes a slower rise in glucose.

Good sources of soluble fiber: Oatmeal… barley, beans (such as kidney, lima and black) and peas…apples, raisins, oranges and bananas…cauliflower and sweet potatoes.

Protein is another natural blood sugar stabilizer—it helps slow the absorption of carbohydrates in your diet. Pairing protein with soluble fiber at every meal will help keep your blood sugar as steady as possible.

Good sources of lean protein: Turkey or chicken breast…fish…pork tenderloin…lean beef…egg whites…yogurt (low-fat or fat-free)…milk (low-fat or fat-free)…and beans (legumes).

My favorite mood-stabilizing combos: Three-bean turkey chili with pinto, black and kidney beans…plain, low-fat or fat-free yogurt with fresh fruit (such as berries)…pork tenderloin with sweet potatoes and cauliflower… hard-boiled eggs with turkey bacon and fruit…and oatmeal with a hard-boiled egg.

Drink Vegetable Juice to Lose Weight

Researchers at Baylor School of Medicine studied overweight adults who had metabolic syndrome, a constellation of risk factors for heart disease and diabetes (such as high blood sugar, high blood pressure and high triglycerides). One group of participants drank at least eight ounces of low-sodium vegetable juice daily for 12 weeks as part of a calorie-restricted diet…a second group followed the same diet but did not drink the juice.

Results: Participants assigned to the vegetable juice group lost four pounds, on average —compared with a loss of only one pound, on average, for the no-juice group.

More research is needed…but in the meantime, drinking vegetable juice on a regular basis can't hurt and may help you meet the goal of increasing vegetable intake while reducing your appetite.

Carl L. Keen, PhD, is a professor of nutrition and internal medicine at the University of California, Davis, and coinvestigator of a study of 81 people.

Nutrient-Boosting Food Combinations

Lisa R. Young, PhD, RD, adjunct professor of nutrition at New York University and a dietitian in private practice, both in New York City. She is author of *The Portion Teller Plan: The No Diet Reality Guide to Eating, Cheating and Losing Weight Permanently* (Broadway), *www.portionteller.com.*

Good nutrition depends not only on what you eat, but also on how well your body absorbs or uses vitamins and minerals in your food. Some nutrients are best absorbed or utilized when consumed with certain other nutrients. Here are easy dishes that combine complementary foods for a synergistic nutritional bonanza—and taste great.

BOOST BETA-CAROTENE TO…

•**Provide antioxidants that protect cells from harmful free radicals.**

•**Enhance immune function.**

Eat with polyunsaturated fat to…

•**Support cognitive function.**

•**Fight inflammation.**

Easy steps for beta-carotene and polyunsaturated fat…

•**Steam sliced butternut squash or carrots** just until soft…for polyunsaturated fat, serve the vegetables with tuna or herring.

• **Bake a sweet potato or half an acorn squash**...for polyunsaturated fat, drizzle with flaxseed oil.

BOOST CALCIUM TO...

• **Build bones.**

• **Help control blood pressure.**

Eat with vitamin D to...

• **Strengthen bones and teeth.**

• **Protect against various cancers.**

Easy steps for calcium...

• **Toss together chopped fresh collard greens and shredded Swiss cheese.**

• **Broil salmon or perch** and serve on a bed of spinach or dandelion greens.

For vitamin D...

• **Stir greens and cheese into beaten eggs to make an omelet or a quiche.**

• **Top fish with mushrooms.**

BOOST FOLATE TO...

• **Reduce risk for Alzheimer's disease.**

• **Protect against birth defects.**

Eat with vitamin C to...

• **Neutralize the toxic by-products of fat metabolism.**

• **Improve absorption of iron, needed for red blood cells.**

Easy steps for folate...

• **Make a spinach and asparagus salad.**

• **Cook great northern beans or black-eyed peas.**

For vitamin C...

• **Toss salad with orange slices, strawberries and lemon vinaigrette.**

• **Stir in chopped tomatoes and red or orange bell peppers to the beans.**

BOOST LUTEIN TO...

• **Protect eyesight.**

• **Combat skin cell damage.**

Eat with monounsaturated fat to...

• **Lower cholesterol and blood pressure.**

• **Combat cancer-causing cell damage.**

Easy steps for lutein...

• **Make a salad of romaine lettuce, green peas and hard-boiled egg.**

• **Mix up a fruit medley of sliced peaches, papaya and oranges.**

For monounsaturated fat...

• **Add avocado slices, shredded low-fat mozzarella and olive oil to the salad.**

• **Stir in chopped hazelnuts, slivered almonds and pumpkin seeds to the fruit.**

BOOST POTASSIUM TO...

• **Promote function of nerve and muscle cells.**

• **Maintain normal blood pressure and heart function.**

Eat with magnesium to...

• **Regulate heartbeat and contractions of the muscles.**

• **Strengthen bones.**

Easy steps for potassium...

• **Combine lentils and lima beans.**

• **Toss together dried apricots and dried banana chips**

Easy steps for magnesium...

• **Stir the legumes into quinoa or bulgur.**

• **Add bran cereal, pumpkin seeds and Brazil nuts to dried fruit to make trail mix.**

BOOST ZINC TO...

• **Strengthen the immune system.**

• **Speed wound healing.**

Eat with protein to...

• **Help build and repair body tissues.**

• **Make hormones and body chemicals.**

Easy steps for zinc...

• **Mix wheat germ into enriched breakfast cereal.**

For protein...

• **Top cereal with low-fat yogurt.**

Salads That Will Change The Way You Eat

Mollie Katzen, author or coauthor of 11 books, including the best-selling *Moosewood Cookbook and Mollie Katzen's Recipes: Salads* (both from Ten Speed). She is a member of the Harvard School of Public Health Nutrition Roundtable and was named by *Health* magazine as one of the five "Women Who Changed the Way We Eat."

Really healthful and refreshing salads bear no resemblance to those boring bowlfuls of wilted, nutrient-challenged iceberg. For maximum health benefits and enjoyment, we want salads that are culinary creations—unique blends packed with nutrition and full of textures, colors and flavor, yet simple and speedy to prepare.

Seem like a tall order? Mollie Katzen, author of the famed *Moosewood Cookbook* and member of the Harvard School of Public Health Nutrition Roundtable, has plenty of super salad recipes that fit the bill.

Bonus: Fiber-rich salads are filling, so food cravings are kept in check.

Each of the following recipes makes four to six servings. Try one today—it will forever change the way you think about salad.

KATZEN'S CALIFORNIA WALDORF SALAD

Special health benefits: The yogurt has calcium to strengthen bones…oranges provide vitamin C to support the immune system…and the omega-3 fatty acids in the avocado contribute to a healthy heart and brain.

Salad…
3 medium apples
2 navel oranges, sectioned
1 stalk celery, minced
¼ cup packed raisins or currants
Lettuce leaves
1 cup sliced ripe mango or papaya
1 cup toasted cashew pieces

Dressing…
1 cup plain low-fat yogurt
½ teaspoon grated lemon rind
2 tablespoons lemon juice
1 ripe avocado, mashed
1 tablespoon honey

In a medium-sized bowl, combine apples, oranges, celery and raisins. In a blender or food processor, puree together all dressing ingredients. Pour dressing over apple mixture and toss well. Spoon onto a bed of lettuce leaves. Top with mango or papaya slices and cashews.

MARINATED SWEET POTATO AND BROCCOLI SALAD

Special health benefits: The sweet potatoes are rich in immune-boosting beta-carotene plus vitamin A for healthy skin and eyes…and the walnut oil provides monounsaturated fats for cardiovascular protection.

Note: While this salad is speedy to prepare, it requires several hours refrigeration before serving.

Salad…
3 medium-sized sweet potatoes or yams, peeled
1 large bunch broccoli, cut into small spears
1 green apple, thinly sliced (optional)

Marinade…
½ cup roasted walnut oil or olive oil
1 garlic clove, minced
3 tablespoons lemon juice
2 tablespoons raspberry vinegar or red wine vinegar
1 teaspoon salt
1 tablespoon dry mustard
1 tablespoon honey
Freshly ground black pepper, to taste

Cut the sweet potatoes into quarters, then into thin slices. Steam or boil potatoes until soft, about eight to 10 minutes. In a medium-sized bowl, combine marinade ingredients. Add hot potatoes to marinade and mix gently. Steam broccoli until bright green and just tender, about five minutes. Rinse broccoli under cold water and drain well. Lay broccoli spears on top of potato-marinade mixture. Cover tightly and refrigerate for several hours. About 15 minutes before serving, stir broccoli into potato mixture. Serve garnished with green apple slices, if desired.

BUTTERMILK SPINACH SALAD WITH STRAWBERRIES

Special health benefits: Bone-building benefits come from the calcium in the spinach and the cheese…the strawberries are packed with antioxidant vitamin C.

Salad…
10 ounces fresh spinach leaves, stemmed and chopped
½ pint fresh strawberries, hulled and cut into quarters
¼ cup thinly sliced red onion
3 ounces fresh goat cheese or Feta cheese, crumbled
Freshly ground black pepper, to taste

Dressing…
2 tablespoons balsamic vinegar

4 tablespoons buttermilk
2 tablespoons light-colored honey
¼ teaspoon salt
2 teaspoons finely minced shallots
5 tablespoons extra-virgin olive oil

In a large salad bowl, gently toss spinach, strawberries and onion. Top with crumbled cheese and black pepper. Set aside. In a small bowl, combine all dressing ingredients except the olive oil and whisk until blended. Continue whisking as you drizzle in the olive oil in a slow, steady stream. (If the taste is too sharp, whisk in more oil.) Pour dressing over salad and toss.

MOLLIE'S CAULIFLOWER-CARROT MEDLEY

Special health benefits: Cauliflower, a cruciferous vegetable, has anticancer properties. Try the new purple or orange varieties of cauliflower, which have higher concentrations of antioxidants.

More plusses: Beta-carotene from the carrots...and the heart-healthy properties of garlic.

Ingredients...
2 tablespoons extra-virgin olive oil
4 cups chopped cauliflower, cut into 1-inch florets
3 medium carrots, cut into thin 1½-inch strips
½ teaspoon salt
2 large cloves garlic, minced
2 tablespoons balsamic vinegar
Freshly ground black pepper, to taste
4 fresh basil leaves, cut into strips

In a medium-to-large skillet, warm the olive oil over medium heat. Add cauliflower, carrots and salt and sauté over medium heat until almost tender, about eight to 10 minutes. Stir in garlic and continue to sauté for three minutes. Transfer mixture to a bowl. Stir in vinegar, pepper and basil. This salad can be served warm, cold or at room temperature.

GINGERY MARINATED CHICKPEA SALAD

Special health benefits: Ginger has anti-inflammatory properties...chickpeas are packed with energizing protein plus immune-boosting zinc.

Note: This is another recipe that requires advanced refrigeration.

Ingredients...
5 cups cooked chickpeas
5 tablespoons lemon juice
2 large cloves garlic, minced
2 tablespoons finely minced ginger
2 tablespoons red wine vinegar
½ cup finely minced red onion
1 teaspoon salt
Freshly ground black pepper, to taste

Rinse and drain the chickpeas. In a medium-sized bowl, combine all ingredients and mix well. Cover tightly and refrigerate for at least four hours, stirring periodically. Serve alone... or with lettuce leaves or over rice, if desired.

Delicious Ways to Get More Fruits, Vegetables

Marjorie Fitch-Hilgenberg, PhD, RD, LD, an associate professor and director of the dietetics program at the University of Arkansas, Fayetteville.

Sauces, marinades and sandwich spreads (commonly known as condiments) have long been relegated to the "bad-for-you" category of foods. But it doesn't have to be that way.

Condiments actually can be good for you—if you choose the right ones. When made from fruits and vegetables, condiments can provide essential vitamins, minerals and other antioxidants that help protect the body from chronic diseases, such as arthritis, heart disease and cancer. Combined with a well-balanced diet, healthful condiments can shore up one's total daily intake of fruits and vegetables.

My favorite condiments (made from ingredients available at most grocery stores)...

- **Cranberry relish.** Cranberries are packed with vitamin C and the flavonoids *anthocyanins* and *proanthocyanidins*—a disease-fighting combination that lowers LDL "bad" cholesterol, helps prevent blood clots that cause heart attacks and stroke, and may fight certain cancers, such as oral and esophageal cancers.

Best uses: It makes a delicious spread for turkey, chicken or pork tenderloin sandwiches, or it can be mixed into sauces and marinades (such as barbecue sauce or a spicy citrus marinade) as a tart counterpoint to meat, fish or poultry dishes. Mix cranberry relish with orange juice (enough to create a syruplike consistency) for a delicious glaze on chicken, turkey or pork.

CRANBERRY RELISH

2 pounds fresh cranberries
1 cup sugar or Splenda (a sugar substitute)
3 tablespoons Grand Marnier liqueur or orange juice
1 orange, zested and juiced

Place all the ingredients in the bowl of a food processor, pulse several times to chop cranberries (until chunky) and mix ingredients. Let relish stand at room temperature for 30 minutes to allow flavor to develop. Relish can be made the day before and stored in the refrigerator until served.

• **Curry.** Long used in south Asian cooking, curry (available in powder form or as a sauce) is a mixture of several pungent spices, including turmeric, a perennial herb that has been found to lower blood levels of LDL cholesterol and raise levels of HDL "good" cholesterol. Turmeric contains curcumin, a substance that may slow the progression of Alzheimer's disease.

Best uses: For a spicy kick, sprinkle curry powder on egg salad or on top of baked chicken. Use curry sauce on beef, pork, chicken, fish or shrimp dishes, or to add zip to rice or vegetables.

• **Guacamole.** This Mexican dip combines mashed avocados with tomatoes, onions, spices, lime juice and heart-healthy garlic. Avocados contain nearly 20 vitamins (such as folate and vitamins C and E), minerals (iron and potassium) as well as fiber. Avocados are rich in cholesterol-lowering monounsaturated fat. Avocados also contain phytonutrients, such as the antioxidant lutein, which may promote eye health.

Best uses: On sandwiches (such as turkey or chicken breast), try guacamole as a low-cholesterol alternative to mayonnaise.

GUACAMOLE

3 avocados
2 tablespoons fresh lime juice (juice from one lime)
½ teaspoon salt
½ cup diced onion
2 tablespoons chopped fresh cilantro
2 plum tomatoes, diced
1 clove garlic, minced (about 1 teaspoon)
Ground cayenne pepper, to taste

Cut avocados in half, remove pit. Scoop avocado into a medium bowl. Add lime juice and salt. Mix while mashing avocados. Add onion, cilantro, tomatoes and garlic. Mix. Season with cayenne pepper. Refrigerate for one hour for best flavor, or serve immediately.

• **Mustard.** An excellent source of iron, calcium, zinc, magnesium and niacin, mustard is an incredibly versatile, low-calorie condiment. Mustard also contains protective phytochemicals called *glucosinolates* that research suggests may help fight prostate, esophageal, gastrointestinal and colorectal cancers.

Best uses: Prepared mustards, such as store-bought yellow mustard—and especially coarse-ground, spicy, brown Dijon—are delicious when used on meat sandwiches, as a base for salad dressing or in marinades and sauces for beef or fish, such as salmon or swordfish. Add honey to mustard to create a sweet-and-sour marinade for pork or chicken or a dipping sauce for finger foods. (Start with two tablespoons of honey to one-half cup of mustard, then add more honey to taste.) For an extra kick, add some horseradish to mustard. Wasabi mustard, a hot mustard available at gourmet food shops, is great on beef or on tuna or salmon fillets. (A little goes a long way.)

Caution: People with high blood pressure should limit their consumption of prepared mustard, which generally is high in sodium (about 50 to 120 milligrams [mg] per teaspoon).

WASABI MUSTARD SAUCE

¼ cup rice wine vinegar
3 tablespoons canola oil
2 teaspoons Dijon mustard

1 teaspoon wasabi paste

Mix all ingredients. Try it on flank steak.

• **Yogurt.** Yogurt contains probiotics, the live, beneficial bacteria that occur naturally in the digestive tract. The most common probiotics in yogurt are *Lactobacillus bulgaricus* and *Streptococcus thermophilus*, which studies show improve intestinal function, fight infection, reduce risk for colon cancer, ease symptoms of irritable bowel syndrome and decrease inflammation associated with arthritis.

Best uses: A healthful, low-fat alternative to mayonnaise or sour cream, plain low-fat yogurt also can be used as a tangy sandwich spread if you add just a little mustard. Yogurt can be used in place of heavy cream to thicken a variety of sauces and stews.

TANGY YOGURT MUSTARD DILL SAUCE

1 cup plain low-fat yogurt
3 tablespoons fresh minced parsley
2 tablespoons Dijon mustard
2 tablespoons fresh dill weed
2 to 3 teaspoons fresh lemon juice
⅛ teaspoon ground pepper, preferably white pepper
Salt to taste

Mix all ingredients. Refrigerate 30 minutes or longer before using. Try it on salmon.

Why Go Nuts for Nuts?

Richard D. Mattes, PhD, MPH, RD, is a professor of foods and nutrition at Purdue University in West Lafayette, Indiana. He has published numerous studies on nuts and appetite.

If you've relegated nuts to the "occasional snack" category, it's time to get more creative. Substitute nuts for some or all of the meat in a stir-fry entrée...sprinkle sliced or chopped nuts over vegetables, rice, soup or cereal...add ground nuts to a smoothie or yogurt...dress salads with nut oils...spread nut butter on celery sticks or apple slices.

Why the push for nuts? Because from all corners of the nutrition world, wellness professionals are touting nuts' amazing health benefits. *Recent research shows that eating a moderate amount of nuts on a regular basis may help...*

• **Control weight.** According to Richard D. Mattes, PhD, MPH, RD, a professor of foods and nutrition at Purdue University who has done extensive research on the topic, nut consumption increases your resting energy expenditure, which means that you burn more calories just sitting still than you otherwise would. Also, about 5% to 15% of the calories in nuts are excreted without being absorbed. And nuts' unique combination of protein, fiber, fatty acids and other characteristics quell hunger quickly and for prolonged periods.

• **Prevent heart disease.** Most of the fats in nuts are heart-healthy monounsaturated fats and omega-3 fatty acids that help lower LDL (bad) cholesterol and triglycerides...increase HDL (good) cholesterol...and prevent abnormal heart rhythms. Nuts also contain vitamin E, which inhibits arterial plaque buildup... and *l-arginine*, an amino acid that makes arteries more flexible and less vulnerable to clots.

• **Fight inflammation.** The soluble fiber in nuts appears to increase production of the anti-inflammatory protein *interleukin-4*. Antioxidant vitamin E also eases inflammation.

• **Reduce diabetes risk.** A Harvard study found that women who ate five or more ounces of nuts weekly were almost 30% less likely to get type 2 diabetes than women who rarely or never ate nuts.

Also: Spanish researchers found that nuts were even more effective than olive oil in combating metabolic syndrome, a condition that puts you at risk for diabetes as well as for heart disease.

• **Combat cancer.** Some nuts (including dried Brazil nuts and walnuts) are high in selenium, a mineral associated with a decreased risk for colorectal, skin and lung cancers. In animal studies, walnuts appeared to inhibit breast tumors—perhaps due to their disease-fighting omega-3s and antioxidants.

• **Support brain function.** Evidence suggests that nuts' omega-3s may ease depression and boost thinking and memory by improving neurotransmitter function. Nuts also provide folate—and low levels of this B-vitamin are linked to depression and poor cognition.

NUT TYPES TO TRY

Per ounce, nuts typically have 160 to 200 calories and 13 to 22 grams of fat. Eating 1.5 ounces of nuts per day (a small handful) is enough to provide health-promoting benefits. Nuts naturally contain only a trace of sodium, so they won't wreak havoc with blood pressure, especially if you choose brands with no added salt.

"All types of nuts are good for you, so there's no such thing as a 'best' type of nut," Dr. Mattes emphasized. Still, each type does contain a different mix of nutrients—so for the widest range of benefits, eat a variety. Below are some excellent options and the nutrients that each is especially rich in. Consider…

- **Almonds** for bone-building calcium…and inflammation-fighting vitamin E.
- **Brazil nuts** for cancer-fighting selenium.
- **Cashews** for magnesium, which may prevent heart attacks and hypertension.
- **Hazelnuts** for potassium, which helps normalize blood pressure.
- **Peanuts** for folate, to lower levels of the artery-damaging amino acid *homocysteine.*
- **Pecans** for *beta-sitosterol,* a plant compound that combats cholesterol.
- **Pistachios** for *gamma-tocopherol,* (vitamin E) which may reduce lung cancer risk.
- **Walnuts** for heart-and brain-enhancing *alpha-linolenic acid,* an omega-3 fatty acid.

Breakthrough Research On Beating Arthritis Pain Naturally

Peter Bales, MD, a board-certified orthopedic surgeon and author of *Osteoarthritis: Preventing and Healing Without Drugs* (Prometheus).

Osteoarthritis has long been considered a "wear-and-tear" disease associated with age-related changes that occur within cartilage and bone.

Now: A growing body of evidence shows that osteoarthritis may have a metabolic basis. Poor diet results in inflammatory changes and damage in cartilage cells, which in turn lead to cartilage breakdown and the development of osteoarthritis.

A recent increase in osteoarthritis cases corresponds to similar increases in diabetes and obesity, other conditions that can be fueled by poor nutrition. Dietary approaches can help prevent—or manage—all three of these conditions.

Key scientific evidence: A number of large studies, including many conducted in Europe as well as the US, suggest that a diet emphasizing plant foods and fish can support cartilage growth and impede its breakdown. People who combine an improved diet with certain supplements can reduce osteoarthritis symptoms—and possibly stop progression of the disease.

A SMARTER DIET

By choosing your foods carefully, you can significantly improve the pain and stiffness caused by osteoarthritis. *How to get started…*

- **Avoid acidic foods.** The typical American diet, with its processed foods, red meat and harmful trans-fatty acids, increases acidity in the body. A high-acid environment within the joints increases free radicals, corrosive molecules that both accelerate cartilage damage and inhibit the activity of cartilage-producing cells known as *chondrocytes.*

A Mediterranean diet, which includes generous amounts of fruits, vegetables, whole grains, olive oil and fish, is more alkaline. (The body requires a balance of acidity and alkalinity, as measured on the pH scale.) A predominantly alkaline body chemistry inhibits free radicals and reduces inflammation.

What to do: Eat a Mediterranean-style diet, including six servings daily of vegetables… three servings of fruit…and two tablespoons of olive oil. (The acids in fruits and vegetables included in this diet are easily neutralized in the body.) Other sources of healthful fats include olives, nuts (such as walnuts), canola oil and flaxseed oil or ground flaxseed.

Important: It can take 12 weeks or more to flush out acidic toxins and reduce arthritis symptoms after switching to an alkaline diet.

- **Limit your intake of sugary and processed foods.** Most Americans consume a lot of refined carbohydrates as well as foods and soft drinks sweetened with sugar—all of which damage joints in several ways. For example, sugar causes an increase in *advanced glycation endproducts* (AGEs), protein molecules that bind to collagen (the connective tissue of cartilage and other tissues) and make it stiff and brittle. AGEs also appear to stimulate the production of enzymes that degrade cartilage.

What to do: Avoid processed foods, such as white flour (including cakes, cookies and crackers), white pasta and white rice, as well as soft drinks and fast food. Studies have shown that people who mainly eat foods in their whole, natural forms tend to have lower levels of AGEs and healthier cartilage.

Important: Small amounts of sugar—used to sweeten coffee or cereal, for example—will not significantly increase AGE levels.

- **Get more vitamin C.** More than 10 years ago, the Framingham study found that people who took large doses of vitamin C had a threefold reduction in the risk for osteoarthritis progression.

Vitamin C is an alkalinizing agent due to its anti-inflammatory and antioxidant properties. It blocks the inflammatory effects of free radicals. Vitamin C also decreases the formation of AGEs and reduces the chemical changes that cause cartilage breakdown.

What to do: Take a vitamin C supplement (1,000 milligrams [mg] daily for the prevention of osteoarthritis...2,000 mg daily if you have osteoarthritis).* Also increase your intake of vitamin C–rich foods, such as sweet red peppers, strawberries and broccoli.

- **Drink green tea.** Green tea alone won't relieve osteoarthritis pain, but people who drink green tea and switch to a healthier diet may notice an additional improvement in symptoms. That's because green tea is among the most potent sources of antioxidants, including catechins, substances that inhibit the activity of cartilage-degrading enzymes.

For osteoarthritis, drink one to two cups of green tea daily. (Check with your doctor first if you take any prescription drugs.)

- **Eat fish.** Eat five to six three-ounce servings of omega-3–rich fish (such as salmon, sardines and mackerel) weekly. Omega-3s in such fish help maintain the health of joint cartilage and help curb inflammation. If you would prefer to take a fish oil supplement rather than eat fish, see the recommendation below.

SUPPLEMENTS THAT HELP

Dietary changes are a first step to reducing osteoarthritis symptoms. However, the use of certain supplements also can be helpful.

- **Fish oil.** The two omega-3s in fish—*docosahexaenoic acid* (DHA) and *eicosapentaenoic acid* (EPA)—block chemical reactions in our cells that convert dietary fats into chemical messengers (such as prostaglandins), which affect the inflammatory status of our bodies. This is the same process that's inhibited by nonsteroidal anti-inflammatory drugs (NSAIDs), such as *ibuprofen* (Motrin).

What to do: If you find it difficult to eat the amount of omega-3–rich fish mentioned above, ask your doctor about taking fish oil supplements that supply a total of 1,600 mg of EPA and 800 mg of DHA daily. Look for a "pharmaceutical grade" fish oil product, such as Sealogix, available at FishOilRx.com, 888-966-3423, *www.fishoilrx.com*...or RxOmega-3 Factors at iherb.com, *www.iherb.com.*

If, after 12 weeks, you need more pain relief—or have a strong family history of osteoarthritis—add...

- **Glucosamine, chondroitin and MSM.** The most widely used supplements for osteoarthritis are glucosamine and chondroitin, taken singly or in combination. Most studies show that they work.

Better: A triple combination that contains *methylsulfonylmethane* (MSM) as well as glucosamine and chondroitin. MSM is a sulfur-containing compound that provides the raw

*Check with your doctor before taking any dietary supplements.

material for cartilage regrowth. Glucosamine and chondroitin reduce osteoarthritis pain and have anti-inflammatory properties.

What to do: Take daily supplements of glucosamine (1,500 mg)...chondroitin (1,200 mg)...and MSM (1,500 mg).

Instead of—or in addition to—the fish oil and the triple combination, you may want to take...

• **SAMe.** Like MSM, *S-adenosylmethionine* (SAMe) is a sulfur-containing compound. It reduces the body's production of *TNF-alpha*, a substance that's involved in cartilage destruction. It also seems to increase cartilage production.

In one study, researchers compared SAMe to the prescription anti-inflammatory drug *celecoxib* (Celebrex). The study was double-blind (neither the patients nor the doctors knew who was getting which drug or supplement), and it continued for four months. Initially, patients taking the celecoxib reported fewer symptoms—but by the second month, there was no difference between the two groups.

Other studies have found similar results. SAMe seems to work as well as over-the-counter and/or prescription drugs for osteoarthritis, but it works more slowly. It usually takes at least three months for patients to see effects.

What to do: Start with 200 mg of SAMe daily and increase to 400 mg daily if necessary after a few weeks.

The Anticancer Diet

Timothy C. Birdsall, ND, vice president of integrative medicine for Cancer Treatment Centers of America, a national network of cancer care facilities. Based in Zion, Illinois, he is coauthor of *How to Prevent and Treat Cancer with Natural Medicine* (Riverhead). *www.cancercenter.com.*

Take healthy cells and expose them to a damaging substance—a toxic chemical, tobacco, radiation, a virus or a bacterium—and the result may be a mutation, a permanent change in cell DNA. Expose the cells again, and you get more mutations. Eventually, the healthy cells can turn into cancer cells.

Mutations also can be triggered by breathing, digesting, moving—in other words, living. As part of metabolism, our bodies create harmful molecules called free radicals, which can damage cell DNA, cause mutations and induce cancer.

First line of defense: an anticancer diet.

FREE RADICAL WEAKENERS

To combat free radicals, we need beneficial nutrients known as antioxidants. *How they work...*

A free radical is an unstable molecule that's missing an electron. To stabilize it, an antioxidant donates one of its own electrons, neutralizing the free radical. Problem solved...except now the antioxidant is missing an electron, so it becomes a free radical. This new free radical is less dangerous than the original one, but it still can damage cells. So you need another antioxidant to give up its electron—and so on. *To get enough antioxidants, eat...*

• **A rainbow of produce.** Varied colors of fruits and vegetables come from antioxidant pigments called phytochemicals. Each plant food contains hundreds of phytochemicals in different combinations.

Remember "Roy G. Biv": The old mnemonic for the colors of the rainbow helps you shop for variety. Go for red raspberries, cranberries, tomatoes...orange pumpkin, papayas, yams...yellow peppers, pineapple, corn... green grapes, asparagus, kale...blue, indigo and violet blueberries, plums and eggplant.

• **Green tea.** These leaves contain antioxidants called *flavonoids.* Consuming green tea daily may reduce risk for various cancers, including bladder and pancreatic cancers.

Recommended: Decaffeination removes flavonoids, so opt for regular green tea rather than decaf. Aim for at least three cups daily, or take green tea extract capsules.

ESTROGEN CONNECTION

The hormone estrogen affects many body functions, including menstruation and cognition. It also may promote some types of breast, ovarian and uterine cancers, although the exact mechanisms are not known. *Protective foods include...*

• **Cruciferous vegetables.** After being used by the body, estrogen is broken down and excreted. The breakdown produces two metabolites, or chemical compounds—one that promotes breast cancer and one that does not. Cruciferous vegetables contain the phytochemical *indole-3-carbinol* (I3C), which promotes formation of estrogen's harmless metabolite instead of its carcinogenic one.

I3C foods: Cabbage, broccoli, cauliflower, kale, brussels sprouts. Have four or five half-cup servings weekly.

• **Soy foods.** Soy contains phytoestrogens (compounds that mimic natural estrogen in the body), including *isoflavones.*

Paradox: Some test-tube studies indicate that concentrated phytoestrogens promote breast cancer cell growth—but in real life, soy seems to protect against breast cancer. In Japan and China, where the typical diet is rich in soy isoflavones, breast cancer incidence is about one-third of the US rate.

Theory: Lifelong intake of isoflavones may reduce natural estrogen levels in breast tissue.

Isoflavone sources: Soy milk, tofu, miso (soybean paste), tempeh (soybean cake), edamame (green soybeans), soy nuts (roasted soybeans).

Goal: One cup of soy milk or one-half cup of another soy food daily.

Caution: Limit soy foods to three servings weekly if you have a history of breast cancer, or are pregnant or nursing. Women with thyroid problems should consult their doctors before eating soy.

• **Fiber.** Estrogen metabolites and toxins pass through the colon on their way out of the body. If they linger there, they can be reabsorbed by the body and cause damage. Fiber may bind to estrogen metabolites and toxins, so they are excreted before they can be reabsorbed.

Goal: Five or more servings per day.

Good sources: Whole-grain bread (one slice) or cereal (typically three-quarters of a cup)...fruit (one piece or one-half cup)...vegetables and legumes (one-half cup)...nuts and seeds (one-quarter cup).

INFLAMMATION FIGHTERS

Inflammation is part of the normal healing process. However, when this mechanism does not turn itself off properly, inflammation becomes chronic.

Result: More free radicals and cell damage that can lead to cancer. *To reduce inflammation, eat...*

• **Fish.** Many fish are rich in beneficial omega-3 fatty acids. Omega-3s contain an inflammation-fighting component called *eicosapentaenoic acid* (EPA). They also create substances called prostaglandins that further reduce inflammation.

Best: Three four-ounce servings weekly of cold-water fatty fish, such as salmon, mackerel, herring and sardines.

Alternative: Take fish oil supplements that provide 1,500 milligrams daily of combined EPA and *docosahexaenoic acid* (DHA).

• **Flaxseeds.** Ground flaxseeds also provide anti-inflammatory omega-3s.

Bonus: Flaxseeds contain compounds called *lignans* that may kill some types of cancer cells.

Smart: Add one tablespoon of ground flaxseeds to your daily diet. Sprinkle on cereal or salad, or add to a fruit smoothie.

• **Turmeric.** This yellow spice, commonly used in curry, contains curcumin, a compound that neutralizes free radicals and shuts down proteins that promote an abnormal inflammatory response.

Use liberally: Sprinkle turmeric on pasta and rice...add it to fish...stir into soups and salad dressings.

Natural Ways to Save Your Sight

Marc Grossman, OD, LAc, an optometrist and licensed acupuncturist who cofounded Integral Health Associates, a private practice in New Paltz, New York, *www.naturaleyecare.com*. A holistic eye doctor with training in Chinese medicine and naturopathic medicine, he is coauthor of *Greater Vision* (McGraw-Hill).

Family history is an uncontrollable risk factor for certain eye diseases. But there are other risk factors for such eye problems as cataracts and macular degeneration that can be minimized with the right nutrition and lifestyle strategies.*

FOLLOW A "VISION CARE" DIET

The most common eye diseases share a common link—oxidation, a chemical process in which disease-causing free radicals damage cells in the body, in this case, eye tissues.

A natural by-product of metabolism, these oxygen-based molecules are also produced in large amounts because of smoking and exposure to air pollution or excessive sunlight.

What helps: An antioxidant-rich diet. A recent study found that women (age 56 to 71) who took supplemental vitamin C for more than 10 years were 77% less likely to develop cataracts than those who didn't take vitamin C.

My advice: Take 250 milligrams (mg) to 500 mg of vitamin C twice daily to protect your eyes, especially against cataracts and macular degeneration (dividing the dose improves absorption).

Caution: If you have hemochromatosis (a disorder marked by excessive absorption and storage of iron in the body), don't take vitamin C supplements—vitamin C increases the amount of iron absorbed from foods. *Also crucial for eye health...*

- **Vitamin A** improves night vision and enhances the ability of the eyes to adapt to changes in light—when you walk from bright sunlight into a dark room, for example. Vitamin A also improves chronic dry eyes.

My advice: Get at least 15 mg of beta-carotene daily (which is converted to vitamin A in the body). People who take a multivitamin and also eat several daily servings of orange- or yellow-pigmented vegetables, including sweet potatoes, carrots and peppers, will get enough beta-carotene and vitamin A to provide substantial eye protection. Smokers should not take beta-carotene supplements—some evidence suggests that they may increase lung cancer risk.

- **Zinc** is an antioxidant mineral that can help prevent night blindness as well as macular degeneration. Take 30 mg of zinc daily in supplement form.
- **Lutein** is an antioxidant that is chemically related to beta-carotene. It reduces eye inflammation induced by ultraviolet radiation from the sun. A Harvard study found that people who consumed about 6 mg of lutein daily (roughly the amount in one-quarter cup of spinach) were 43% less likely to develop macular degeneration than those who consumed less. People who eat a lot of spinach and other green, leafy vegetables can reduce the risk for cataracts by up to 50%.

My advice: Eat at least one-quarter cup of spinach, kale or collard greens daily.

- **Fish oil** contains *docosahexaenoic acid* (DHA), an omega-3 fatty acid that repairs damage to cell membranes in the eyes. It improves eye circulation and also seems to help people with chronic dry eyes.

My advice: To ensure adequate intake of DHA, take 1,000 mg of purified fish oil liquid or gels (the most absorbable forms) twice daily. Purified fish oil contains no contaminants such as mercury.

Recommended brands: Nordic Naturals Omega-3, 800-662-2544, *www.nordicnaturals.com*...or J.R. Carlson Laboratories, Inc., Very Finest Fish Oil, 888-234-5656, *www.carlsonlabs.com*.

WATER AND EXERCISE

Drinking a lot of fluids improves the transport of antioxidant nutrients to eye tissues.

My advice: Drink at least eight glasses of water a day to lubricate the eyes.

Regular exercise also is good for eye health—especially in helping to prevent glaucoma. It boosts circulation throughout the body (including the eyes) and can reduce pressure within the

*Consult your doctor before beginning any supplement regimen, including the one in this article.

eye by about 2.5 mm (normal range is 10 mm to 22 mm). That's about the same reduction you would get from using beta-blocker eyedrops, which are commonly prescribed for glaucoma.

My advice: Take a brisk, 40-minute walk most days of the week.

DON'T FORGET SUNGLASSES

Most people wear sunglasses for comfort or to prevent eye wrinkles. But there's a more important reason—the sun's ultraviolet radiation greatly increases oxidation in eye tissues. Excessive sun exposure is a leading cause of cataracts and macular degeneration.

My advice: Except when it's raining, always wear sunglasses when you go outside during the day, even on cloudy days. Buy sunglasses that block 100% of both UVA and UVB radiation. The wraparound styles are ideal as this design blocks most of the sunlight that would otherwise hit your eyes.

RELAX YOUR EYES

Except when we're asleep, our eyes get virtually no rest.

My advice: At least once daily, rub your palms together briskly until they're warm. Cup your hands and place the base of the palms gently over your closed eyes with the fingers of each hand overlapping and resting gently in the center of the forehead for a few minutes. This helps soothe and relax your eyes.

You Can Cure Heart Disease—with Plant-Based Nutrition

Caldwell B. Esselstyn, Jr., MD, surgeon, clinician and researcher at The Cleveland Clinic for more than 35 years. He is author of *Prevent and Reverse Heart Disease.* (Avery). *www.heartattackproof.com.*

In the mid-1980s, 17 people with severe heart disease had just about given up hope. They had undergone every available treatment, including drugs and surgery—all had failed. The group had experienced 49 cardiovascular events, including four heart attacks, three strokes, 15 cases of increased angina and seven bypass surgeries. Five of the patients were expected to die within a year.

Twelve years later, every one of the 17 was alive. They had had no cardiovascular events. The progression of their heart disease had been stopped—and, in many cases, reversed. Their angina went away—for some, within three weeks. In fact, they became virtually heart-attack proof. And there are hundreds of other patients with heart disease who have achieved the same remarkable results. *What you need to know...*

HOW THE DAMAGE IS DONE

Every year, more than half a million Americans die of coronary artery disease (CAD). Three times that number suffer heart attacks. In total, half of American men and one-third of women will have some form of heart disease during their lifetimes.

Heart disease develops in the *endothelium,* the lining of the arteries. There, endothelial cells manufacture a compound called nitric oxide that accomplishes four tasks crucial for healthy circulation...

- **Keeps blood smoothly flowing,** rather than becoming sticky and clotted.
- **Allows arteries to widen when the heart needs more blood,** such as when you run up a flight of stairs.
- **Stops muscle cells in arteries from growing into plaque**—the fatty gunk that blocks blood vessels.
- **Decreases inflammation in the plaque**—the process that can trigger a rupture in the cap or surface of a plaque, starting the clot-forming, artery-clogging cascade that causes a heart attack.

The type and amount of fat in the typical Western diet—from animal products, dairy foods and concentrated oils—assaults endothelial cells, cutting their production of nitric oxide.

Study: A researcher at University of Maryland School of Medicine fed a 900-calorie fast-food breakfast containing 50 grams of fat (mostly from sausages and hash browns) to a group of students and then measured their endothelial function. For six hours, the students had severely compromised endothelial function and decreased nitric oxide production. Another group ate a 900-calorie, no-fat breakfast—and had no significant change in endothelial function.

If a single meal can do that kind of damage, imagine the damage done by three fatty meals a day, seven days a week, 52 weeks a year.

PLANT-BASED NUTRITION

You can prevent, stop or reverse heart disease with a plant-based diet. *Here's what you can't eat—and what you can...*

What you cannot eat...

- **No meat, poultry, fish or eggs.** You will get plenty of protein from plant-based sources.
- **No dairy products.** That means no butter, cheese, cream, ice cream, yogurt or milk—even skim milk, which, though lower in fat, still contains animal protein.
- **No oil of any kind**—not a drop. That includes all oils, even virgin olive oil and canola.

What you may not know: At least 14% of olive oil is saturated fat—every bit as aggressive in promoting heart disease as the saturated fat in roast beef. A diet that includes oils—including monounsaturated oils from olive oil and canola oil—may slow the progression of heart disease, but it will not stop or reverse the disease.

- **Generally, no nuts or avocados.** If you are eating a plant-based diet to prevent heart disease, you can have moderate amounts of nuts and avocados as long as your total cholesterol remains below 150 milligrams per deciliter (mg/dL). If you have heart disease and want to stop or reverse it, you should not eat these foods.

What you can eat...

- **All vegetables.**
- **Legumes**—beans, peas, lentils.
- **Whole grains** and products that are made from them, such as bread and pasta—as long as they do not contain added fats. Do not eat refined grains, which have been stripped of much of their fiber and nutrients. Avoid white rice and "enriched" flour products, which are found in many pastas, breads, bagels and baked goods.
- **Fruits**—but heart patients should limit consumption to three pieces a day and avoid drinking pure fruit juices. Too much fruit rapidly raises blood sugar, triggering a surge of insulin from the pancreas—which stimulates the liver to manufacture more cholesterol.
- **Certain beverages, including water, seltzer water, oat milk, hazelnut milk, almond milk, no-fat soy milk, coffee and tea.** Alcohol is fine in moderation (no more than two servings a day for men and one for women).

SUPPLEMENTS TO TAKE

For maximum health, take five supplements daily...

- **Multivitamin/mineral supplement.**
- **Vitamin B-12**—1,000 micrograms (mcg).
- **Calcium**—1,000 milligrams (mg) (1,200 mg if you're over 60).
- **Vitamin D-3**—1,000 international units (IU).
- **Flaxseed meal** (ground flaxseed)—one tablespoon for the omega-3 fatty acids it provides. Sprinkle it on cereal.

THE CHOLESTEROL CONNECTION

If you eat the typical, high-fat Western diet, even if you also take a cholesterol-lowering statin drug, you will not protect yourself from heart disease—because the fat in the diet will damage the endothelium cells that produce nitric oxide.

In a study in *The New England Journal of Medicine*, patients took huge doses of statin drugs to lower total cholesterol below 150 but didn't change their diets—and 25% experienced a new cardiovascular event or died within the next 30 months.

Recommended: Eat a plant-based diet, and ask your doctor if you should also take a cholesterol-lowering medication. Strive to maintain a total cholesterol of less than 150 and LDL ("bad" cholesterol) below 85.

MODERATION DOESN'T WORK

The most common objection physicians have to this diet is that their patients will not follow it. But many patients with heart disease who find out that they have a choice—between invasive surgery and nutritional changes that will stop and reverse the disease—willingly adopt the diet.

Why not eat a less demanding diet, such as the low-fat diet recommended by the American Heart Association or the Mediterranean Diet?

Surprising: Research shows that people who maintain a so-called low-fat diet of 29% of calories from fat have the same rate of heart attacks and strokes as people who don't.

Plant-based nutrition is the only diet that can effectively prevent, stop and reverse heart disease. It also offers protection against stroke...high blood pressure...osteoporosis...diabetes...senile mental impairment...erectile dysfunction...and cancers of the breast, prostate, colon, rectum, uterus and ovaries.

The Real Secret to Strong Bones

Susan E. Brown, PhD, medical anthropologist, certified nutritionist and director, The Center for Better Bones and Better Bones Foundation, both in Syracuse, New York. She is author of *Better Bones, Better Body* (McGraw-Hill) and *The Acid-Alkaline Food Guide* (Square One). *www.betterbones.com.*

Contrary to popular belief, the degenerative bone disease osteoporosis is not an inevitable result of aging. New research is showing that an important but overlooked cause of osteoporosis is an acid-forming diet.

Susan E. Brown, PhD, is author of *Better Bones, Better Body. Her insights into this important research...*

THE ACID/ALKALI BALANCE

For survival, the body must maintain a balance between acids and alkalis, with good health depending on slight alkalinity. If the body's alkali reserves run low—a condition called chronic low-grade metabolic acidosis—alkaline mineral compounds are drawn from bones to buffer excess acids in the blood. The immediate benefit is that the body's pH (a measure of acidity or alkalinity) is balanced. But over time, if bone mineral compounds are not replenished, osteoporosis develops.

Bone-depleting metabolic acidosis is easily reversible through diet. Yet the average American diet is woefully deficient in many of the nutrients needed to balance pH.

To protect bones: Follow the dietary suggestions on the next page. It's generally best to get nutrients from food. However, to help ensure adequate intake, take a daily multivitamin/mineral plus the other supplements noted...and consider additional supplements as well.

Before you start: Gauge your pH with a urine test kit, such as those sold in some pharmacies...or use the Better Bones Alkaline for Life pH Test Kit.

Cost: $29.95 (*www.betterbones.com*, click on "Visit Our Store," or call 888-206-7119). An ideal first morning urine pH is 6.5 to 7.5. The lower your pH is, the more helpful supplements may be. As with any supplement regimen, talk to your doctor before beginning.

BONE-SUPPORTIVE DIET

For a diet that builds bones...

- **Emphasize vegetables** (particularly dark, leafy greens and root vegetables), fruits, nuts, seeds and spices—these are alkalizing.

Daily targets: Eight servings of vegetables...three to four servings of fruit...two servings of nuts or seeds...and plentiful spices.

- **Consume meat, poultry, fish, dairy, eggs, legumes and whole grains in moderation—** they are acidifying.

Daily targets: One serving of meat, poultry or fish...one serving of eggs or legumes...one to two servings each of dairy and whole grains.

- **Minimize sugar, refined grains and processed foods...**limit coffee to two servings daily...limit alcohol to one serving daily. All these are very acidifying.

- **Fats neither increase nor decrease blood acidity—but for overall health, keep fat intake moderate** and opt for those that protect the heart, such as olive oil.

Important: It's not the acidity of a food itself that matters, but rather its metabolic effects. For instance, citrus fruits taste acidic, yet once metabolized, they are alkalizing.

MINERALS THAT BONES NEED MOST

Bone is composed of a living protein matrix of collagen upon which mineral crystals are deposited in a process called mineralization. Key minerals, in order of importance...

• **Potassium** neutralizes metabolic acids and reduces calcium loss.

Daily goal: 4,000 milligrams (mg) to 6,000 mg.

Sources: Avocados, baked potatoes, bananas, beet greens, cantaloupe, lima beans, sweet potatoes.

• **Magnesium** boosts absorption of calcium and production of the bone-preserving hormone *calcitonin.*

Daily goal: 400 mg to 800 mg.

Sources: Almonds, Brazil nuts, kelp, lentils, pumpkin seeds, soy, split peas, whole wheat, wild rice.

• **Calcium** gives bones strength.

Daily goal: 1,000 mg to 1,500 mg.

Sources: Amaranth flour, broccoli, canned sardines with bones, collards, dairy, kale, mustard greens, sesame seeds, spinach.

Also: Supplement daily, at a two-to-one ratio, with calcium citrate or calcium citrate malate plus magnesium—increasing calcium intake without also increasing magnesium can exacerbate asthma, arthritis and kidney stones.

• **Zinc** aids collagen production and calcium absorption.

Daily goal: 20 mg to 30 mg.

Sources: Alaskan king crab, cashews, kidney beans, meat, oysters, sesame seeds, wheat germ.

• **Manganese** helps form bone cartilage and collagen.

Daily goal: 10 mg to 15 mg.

Sources: Beets, blackberries, brown rice, loganberries, oats, peanuts, pineapple, rye, soy.

• **Copper** blocks bone breakdown and increases collagen formation.

Daily goal: 1 mg to 3 mg.

Sources: Barley, beans, chickpeas, eggplant, liver, molasses, summer squash.

• **Silica** increases collagen strength and bone calcification.

Daily goal: 30 mg to 50 mg.

Sources: Bananas, carrots, green beans, whole grains.

• **Boron** helps the body use calcium, magnesium and vitamin D.

Daily goal: 3 mg to 5 mg.

Sources: Almonds, avocados, black-eyed peas, cherries, grapes, tomatoes.

• **Strontium** promotes mineralization.

Daily goal: 3 mg to 20 mg.

Sources: Brazil nuts, legumes, root vegetables, whole grains.

VITAL VITAMINS

The following vitamins enhance bones' self-repair abilities...

• **Vitamin D** is essential because, without adequate amounts, you cannot absorb enough calcium. Many people do not get adequate vitamin D from sunlight. Vitamin D deficiency accounts for up to 50% of osteoporotic fractures.

Daily goal: 1,000 international units (IU) to 2,000 IU.

Best source: A daily supplement of cholecalciferol (vitamin D-3)—foods that contain vitamin D (fatty fish, fortified milk) do not provide enough and are acidifying.

• **Vitamins K-1 and K-2** boost bone matrix synthesis and bind calcium and phosphorous to bone.

Daily goal: 1,000 micrograms (mcg) of K-1...and 90 mg to 180 mg of K-2.

Sources: Aged cheese, broccoli, Brussels sprouts, collard greens, kale, spinach, green tea.

If you supplement: For vitamin K-2, choose the MK-7 form.

Caution: Vitamin K can interfere with blood thinners, such as warfarin (Coumadin)—so talk to your doctor before altering vitamin K intake.

• **Vitamin C** aids collagen formation, stimulates bone-building cells and helps synthesize the adrenal hormones vital to postmenopausal bone health.

Daily goal: 500 mg to 2,000 mg.

Sources: Cantaloupe, kiwifruit, oranges, papaya, pink grapefruit, red peppers, strawberries.

• **Vitamins B-6, B-12 and folate** help eliminate homocysteine, an amino acid linked to fracture risk.

Daily goal: 25 mg to 50 mg of B-6...200 mcg to 800 mcg of B-12...800 mcg to 1,000 mcg of folate.

Sources: For B-6—avocados, bananas, brown rice, oats, turkey, walnuts. For B-12—beef, salmon, trout. For folate—asparagus, okra, peanuts, pinto beans.

• **Vitamin A** helps develop bone-building osteoblast cells.

Daily goal: 5,000 IU.

Sources: Carrots, collard greens, pumpkin, sweet potatoes.

If you supplement: Choose the supplement with the beta-carotene form.

SPECIAL REPORT #5

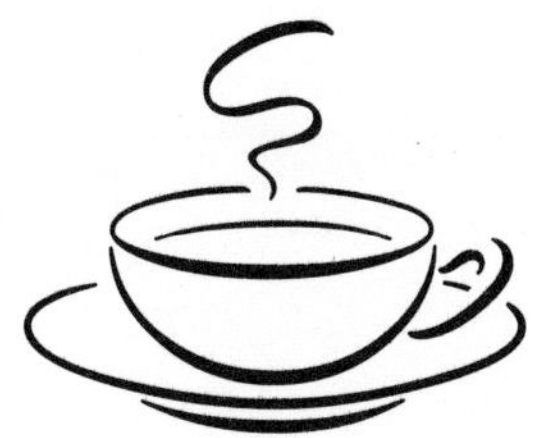

The Truth About Vitamins & Supplements: The Lifesavers & the Money Wasters

The Truth About Vitamins & Supplements: The Lifesavers & the Money Wasters

Best Supplements for Healthy Aging

Of all the changes that occur with aging, one of the most under-recognized is the body's reduced ability to absorb nutrients. As we grow older, our bodies become less efficient at secreting the digestive enzymes that are necessary for the absorption of essential vitamins. Because of this absorption problem, I advise my older patients to follow the nutritious and heart-healthy Mediterranean diet—rich in fresh greens (such as chard, kale and spinach), fresh fruit, whole grains, nuts, seeds, beans, healthful oils (olive, for example) and lean protein, such as turkey and fish. For more on the Mediterranean diet, visit the Web site of the American Heart Association, *www.heart.org*.

But it's not always easy to stick to a nutritious eating plan. What's more, many older adults suffer conditions that interfere with appetite—for example, dry mouth, nausea or constipation caused by common medications, such as pain relievers and hypertension drugs. Dentures and waning senses of smell and taste also can interfere with the consumption of healthful meals. In my opinion, all people over age 50 should consider taking certain supplements—in addition to a daily multivitamin—to compensate for nutrients that might be lacking in their diets. *My favorite "healthy aging" supplements (all available at health-food stores)...*

- **Vitamin B-12**—800 micrograms (mcg) to 1,000 mcg daily, in sublingual (dissolved under the tongue) form. It helps with poor memory, a lack of energy, depression and neuralgia (nerve pain).
- **Vitamin A**—10,000 international units (IU) daily. It helps promote health of the eyes and skin and general immunity. If you also take a multivitamin containing vitamin A, do not

Jamison Starbuck, ND, a naturopathic physician in family practice, Missoula, Montana. She is past president of the American Association of Naturopathic Physicians and a contributing editor to *The Alternative Advisor: The Complete Guide to Natural Therapies and Alternative Treatments* (Time-Life).

exceed 10,000 IU daily unless recommended by your doctor.

• **Vitamin E**—400 IU daily. It protects nerve and muscle cells, reduces leg cramps and helps prevent heart disease.*

• **Vitamin D**—1,000 IU daily. Recent research shows that many older adults are deficient in vitamin D, a nutrient that is essential for calcium absorption and osteoporosis prevention and may protect against certain malignancies, including cancers of the breast and colon.

• **Essential fatty acids,** in the form of fish oil, containing 1,800 milligrams (mg) daily of combined *eicosapentaenoic acid* (EPA) and *docosahexaenoic acid* (DHA). Fish oil acts as a natural antidepressant for patients of all ages and improves brain function.

• **Digestive enzymes.** Typically derived from papaya or pineapple, digestive enzyme supplements promote digestion—and, in turn, the absorption of nutrients from foods and other supplements. Follow the manufacturer's directions for dosages. If you have a gastrointestinal disease, such as an ulcer or diverticulitis, consult your physician before taking plant enzymes, which can irritate an inflamed gastrointestinal tract.

*If you take a blood-thinning drug, such as *warfarin* (Coumadin), check with your doctor before taking vitamin E supplements.

The Most Common Vitamin Deficiencies

Andrew L. Rubman, ND, consulting medical editor, *Daily Health News*, and director, Southbury Clinic for Traditional Medicines, Southbury, Connecticut.

Office of Dietary Supplements, National Institutes of Health, *http://ods.od.nih.gov*.

There seems to be a few key vitamins and minerals that are critical to vibrant health and yet most people tend to be lacking in them. According to *Daily Health News* consulting medical editor Andrew L. Rubman, ND, these deficiencies can hit even people with the most healthful of diets, because diet alone is often insufficient to provide enough of these vitamins and minerals to meet a person's needs. In these cases supplements come into play, but often at different levels than the government-recommended Daily Value (DV) or Recommended Dietary Allowance (RDA), which are not necessarily the levels for optimal health. This is particularly true about vitamin B-12, calcium, magnesium and iron, said Dr. Rubman.

VITAMIN B-12: ESSENTIAL TO PROPER LIVER FUNCTION

One of the most common deficiencies of all is B-12, which the liver requires for optimal function in a myriad of roles including nutrient synthesis and transportation, and waste management and selective recycling, says Dr. Rubman. He notes that older people, in particular, are very often functionally deficient in B-12. The truth is that normal government-recommended values are based on vulnerability to pernicious anemia (a type of anemia caused by extreme B-12 deficiency) rather than reflective of individual needs. While most people don't develop this severe type of anemia, a significant percentage of the population has a functional deficiency such that they are unable to operate at an optimal level. Given how essential B-12 is to brain and nervous system function, a functional deficiency can lead to neurological issues. Problems such as impaired memory, confusion and decreased cognition may seem subtle at first, but if the deficiency is not addressed, over time these problems may grow more pronounced. In older people, a B-12 deficiency is one contributing factor to dementia. This is why they must seek professional oversight.

What you can do: Dr. Rubman encourages people to get a serum blood test to assess their level of B-12. If there is a functional deficiency, he recommends sublingual B-12 pills, either *hydroxocobalamin* or *methylcobalamin*, which are equally as effective as and less expensive than B-12 shots. (Avoid *cyanocobalamin*, which is poorly absorbed.) B-12 should be taken under a doctor's supervision. Because B-12 requires other B vitamins to function properly in the body, take a multi-B supplement twice daily, as they do not last 24 hours in circulation.

Note: Take B-12 and a multi-B supplement under the supervision of your physician. A good way to know if you're taking in sufficient B is to look at the color of your urine. Ideally, it should remain yellow through the day.

CALCIUM AND MAGNESIUM: FOR BONE HEALTH AND MORE

Calcium is the most abundant mineral in the body, required for bone formation and for maintaining strong bones throughout life as well as for assisting in sleep and blood clotting. Insufficient calcium can lead to the bone-thinning disorders osteoporosis and osteopenia. While dairy products are the most popular sources of calcium, cow's milk is difficult to digest and may not be the best form of calcium for absorption. Other sources you may want to try are calcium-enriched plant milks (e.g., almond, oat, hazelnut, rice and soy) and leafy green vegetables such as spinach and kale.

Magnesium, the fourth most abundant mineral in the body, is required to ensure calcium absorption as well as proper muscle and nerve function, bone strength and to keep heart rhythm steady. Many people do not take in enough magnesium (through foods such as legumes, nuts, whole grains and vegetables), which is believed to offer protection against cardiovascular disease and immune dysfunction. Gastrointestinal disorders such as insufficient stomach acid or Crohn's disease may impair the absorption of magnesium.

What you can do: Dr. Rubman often prescribes calcium and magnesium in the combination supplement Butyrex, made by T.E. Neesby. These capsules contain calcium/magnesium as *butyrates*, a form which makes them much easier for the body to absorb than that found in other commonly available supplements. Butyrex has a number of gastrointestinal benefits. It supports the lining of the gastrointestinal tract, allowing for optimal absorption of nutrients, and helps maintain a balanced microbial population in the gut. While the standard RDA for calcium is 800 to 1,200 milligrams (mg) per day along with magnesium in a 2:1 proportion, Butyrex's formulation is so well absorbed that the dosing is often lower. According to Dr. Rubman, patients often start feeling better within just a few days of taking Butyrex.

IRON: FOR OXYGEN TRANSPORT AND ENERGY

Iron is a tricky nutrient. According to the World Health Organization, iron deficiency is the most common nutritional deficiency in the world, with as many as 80% of the global population suffering from iron deficiency or iron deficiency anemia. On the other hand, too much iron can also cause problems, warns Dr. Rubman.

If you don't take in enough iron, oxygen is not transported efficiently to the body's cells. As a result, you're apt to feel tired and weak, and be more susceptible to infection. Women with heavy menstrual periods are at risk for iron deficiency, as are pregnant women, children and teens, all of whom have a high need for iron. Gastrointestinal disorders such as Crohn's disease, celiac disease, ulcers and other GI disorders, as well as the chronic use of antacids and acid suppressing medications, may impair the absorption of iron.

What you can do: Dietary sources of iron include animal proteins such as red meat, turkey, chicken and fish. Other sources include lentils, soybeans, kidney beans, spinach and enriched breads and cereals. If needed, it is fine to take iron as part of a multivitamin supplement, says Dr. Rubman. Otherwise, he recommends taking the superior iron supplement Proferrin, only under medical supervision.

The Most Powerful Brain-Building Nutrients And Herbs

Maoshing Ni ("Dr. Mao"), PhD, DOM (doctor of oriental medicine), LAc (licensed acupuncturist), chancellor and cofounder of Yo San University in Los Angeles, and codirector of Tao of Wellness, a clinic in Santa Monica, California. He is author of numerous books, including *Second Spring: Dr. Mao's Hundreds of Natural Secrets for Women to Revitalize and Regenerate at Any Age* (Free Press). *www.taoofwellness.com.*

You open your cupboard but then can't recall what you wanted...you're introducing two friends and suddenly draw a blank on one's name.

Such instances of "brain fog" are common, but they are not an inevitable part of aging. Many people remain remarkably sharp all their lives—and the right nutritional strategies can help you be one of them.

Cognitive declines can result from hormonal changes and reductions in neurotransmitters, chemicals that help brain cells communicate with each other. Increasing your intake of certain nutrients helps balance hormones and protect neurotransmitters. *You can get these nutrients from...*

• **Foods.** Eating brain-boosting foods is an ideal way to get needed nutrients.

Reasons: The body is designed to absorb nutrients from foods rather than from isolated or manufactured chemicals (such as in supplements)...and foods contain complementary components that enhance nutrient absorption.

• **Herbs.** The healthful aromatic oils are most active when herbs are fresh, but dried herbs also will do.

• **Supplements.** These are an option if you cannot find the foods that provide certain nutrients, or if you need specific nutrients in quantities beyond what you typically get from food. Unless otherwise noted, the following supplements generally are safe, have few side effects and may be used indefinitely. All are sold at health-food stores.

Important: Ask your doctor before supplementing, especially if you have a health condition...use medication...or are pregnant or breast-feeding. To reduce the risk for interactions, do not take supplements within 30 minutes of medication...and limit your use of these supplements to any four of the following.

NUTRIENTS YOUR MIND NEEDS

For the foods recommended below, one serving equals four ounces of meat, poultry, fish, or soy products...eight ounces of milk...two ounces of nuts...two eggs (with yolks)...one-half cup of vegetables or fruit...and one cup of leafy greens.

• **Choline.** The neurotransmitter *acetylcholine* plays a key role in learning and memory. Choline is a precursor to acetylcholine that is produced in the liver. Production of choline declines with age, as does the body's ability to efficiently use the choline that remains.

Brain boost: Eat one or more servings daily of choline-rich broccoli, cauliflower, eggs, kidney beans, navy beans, liver, milk or peanuts.

Supplement option: 1,200 milligrams (mg) daily.

• **DMAE (*2-dimethylaminoethanol*).** The body uses fatty acids to create brain cells and neurotransmitters. DMAE, a chemical in fatty acids, helps produce acetylcholine.

Brain boost: Have two servings weekly of DMAE-rich anchovies or sardines. If fresh fish is not available, have canned water-packed sardines or anchovies and rinse before eating to reduce salt.

Supplement option: 500 mg twice daily after meals.

• **L-carnitine.** Mitochondria are the engines of cells. The amino acid L-carnitine transports fatty acids to mitochondria for use as fuel and provides nutrients to brain cells.

Brain boost: Have two weekly servings of lamb or poultry, which are rich in L-carnitine. Supplement option: 500 mg to 1,000 mg before breakfast and again in the afternoon.

Supplement option: 500 mg to 1,000 mg before breakfast and again in the afternoon.

• **Vitamin B-12.** This is key to red blood cell formation and nerve cell health. The body's ability to absorb vitamin B-12 diminishes with age—about 10% to 15% of people over age 60 are deficient in it.

Brain boost: Have two servings weekly of beef or lamb...halibut, salmon, sardines or sea bass...eggs...or vitamin B-12–enriched soybean products (miso, tempeh).

Supplement option: 500 micrograms (mcg) to 1,000 mcg daily.

THE MOST HELPFUL HERBS

An easy way to get the benefits of mind-sharpening herbs is to brew them into a *tisane*, or herbal infusion—more commonly called herbal tea.

To brew: Pour eight ounces of very hot water over one heaping tablespoon of fresh herbs or one teaspoon of dried herbs. Steep for five minutes, strain and drink.

Convenient: To reduce the number of cups needed to meet the daily recommendations below, brew two or more herbs together.

• **Chinese club moss.** This herb contains the chemical huperzine A, which helps conserve acetylcholine.

Brain boost: Drink one to two cups of Chinese club moss tea each day.

Supplement option: 50 mcg of *huperzine A* twice daily (discontinue if supplements cause gastric upset or hyperactivity).

• **Ginkgo biloba.** This herb increases blood flow to the brain's tiny capillaries and combats DNA damage caused by free radicals.

Caution: Do not use ginkgo if you take blood-thinning medication, such as *warfarin* (Coumadin).

Brain boost: Drink three cups of ginkgo tea daily.

Supplement option: 120 mg daily.

• **Kitchen herbs.** Oregano, peppermint, rosemary and sage have oils that may increase blood flow in the brain and/or support neurotransmitters, promoting alertness.

Brain boost: Use any or all of these herbs to brew a cup of tea for a pick-me-up in the morning and again in the afternoon.

Also: Use herbs liberally when cooking.

Supplement option: 150 mg each of any or all of these herbs daily, alone or combined.

• **Mugwort (wormwood).** This herb improves circulation, aiding delivery of nutrients to brain cells.

Brain boost: Twice a week, drink one cup of mugwort tea...add a half-dozen leaves of fresh mugwort to salad...or sauté leaves with garlic or onions.

Supplement option: 300 mg daily.

Caution: Avoid mugwort during pregnancy—it may stimulate uterine contractions.

Don't forget: Green Tea

Strictly speaking, an herb is a flowering plant whose stem above ground does not become woody. In that sense, the leaf of the *Camellia sinensis* shrub—otherwise known as tea—is not an herb. Yet green tea (which is less oxidized than black) is so helpful that it must be listed among the top brain boosters.

Along with antioxidant *polyphenols*, green tea provides the amino acid theanine, which stimulates calming alpha brain waves and improves concentration. Green tea also has been linked to a reduced risk for Alzheimer's disease.

To brew: Pour eight ounces of very hot water over one teaspoon of loose, fresh green tea leaves (or a tea bag if fresh is not available) and steep for three to five minutes. You needn't strain the tea. As you empty your cup, you can add more warm water to the remaining leaves—as long as the water turns green, the tea still contains polyphenols.

Brain boost: Drink three cups of green tea (caffeinated or decaffeinated) daily.

Supplement option: 350 mg of green tea extract daily.

The "Daily Dozen" Supplements for Women

Earl Mindell, RPh, PhD, professor emeritus of nutrition at Pacific Western University in Los Angeles and an internationally recognized expert on vitamins and herbal remedies. He has a private practice in Beverly Hills and is the author or coauthor of more than 50 books, including *Bottom Line's Prescription Alternatives* (Bottom Line Books), and *Earl Mindell's New Vitamin Bible* (Grand Central).

Even women who eat healthfully and take a multivitamin do not always get enough of the following 12 essential nutrients.

Best: Check the label on your multi, then make up for shortfalls with additional supplements. For maximum absorption, take supplements with meals. Supplements that are most effective when taken at the same time are grouped together below. Take the others at your convenience.

Important: Talk to your doctor before beginning supplementation. Some supplements should be avoided or used only under a doctor's supervision by people who take medication or have a medical condition.

TAKE DAILY

Take these together...

- **Calcium.** 1,500 milligrams (mg).

Best form: Calcium citrate.

- Take in three doses—the body can absorb only 500 mg at a time.
- It may decrease the effectiveness of the heart medication *digoxin* (Lanoxin).

- **Magnesium.** 350 mg.

- Taking more than 350 mg a day may worsen kidney problems.

- **Vitamin D.** 800 international units (IU).

Best form: Cholecalciferol (vitamin D-3).

- Increase daily dosage to 1,000 IU if you get little sunshine.
- Do not exceed 2,000 IU daily—this can raise blood calcium levels, increasing risk for digestive, cardiac and cognitive problems.

Take these together...

- **Selenium.** 100 micrograms (mcg).

- Do not exceed 400 mcg daily—this can cause digestive problems as well as skin discoloration.

- **Vitamin A.** 400 IU.

- Use a brand that includes beta-carotene, a vitamin-A precursor.
- If you smoke, do not supplement with vitamin A or beta-carotene, because this may increase lung cancer risk.

- **Vitamin E.** 200 IU.

Best form: Natural d-alpha-tocopherol with gamma-tocopherol.

- It may increase bleeding risk in people who take blood-thinning or anti-inflammatory drugs.
- It may not be appropriate for people deficient in vitamin K.

Take these individually as needed...

- **Vitamin-B Complex.**

B-1, B-2, B-3, B-6, choline: 50 mg each.

Folic acid: 400 mcg.

B-12: 100 mcg.

- Taking just one type of B vitamin can deplete levels of the others, so opt for a combination B-complex supplement.
- B-3 can exacerbate diabetes, gout and liver problems.
- Avoid B-6 if you take L-dopa for Parkinson's disease.

- **Boron.** 3 mg.

- Do not exceed 10 mg daily—this could be toxic.

- **Coenzyme Q10.** 90 mg.

Best form: Oil-based gel.

- It may not be appropriate if you have diabetes or hypoglycemia, because it can lower blood sugar levels.

- **Omega-3 Fatty Acids.** 1,000 mg of EPA/DHA.

Best form: Fish oil or krill oil.

- Do not exceed 3,000 mg—this might cause bruising and/or internal bleeding.
- It may increase bleeding risk in people taking blood thinners.

- **Vitamin C.** 1,000 mg.

- Take in two doses—the body can absorb only 500 mg at a time.
- In excess, it may alter the effects of blood thinners.

- **Vitamin K.** 100 mcg.

- In excess, it may alter the effects of blood thinners.

Ladies, Are You Taking The Right Multivitamin?

Alan H. Pressman, DC, PhD, CCN (certified clinical nutritionist), director of Gramercy Health Associates, New York City. He hosts the radio show *"Healthline"* and is coauthor of *The Complete Idiot's Guide to Vitamins and Minerals* (Alpha).

A daily multivitamin/mineral supplement helps you meet your nutritional needs—but with so many brands available, it's not easy to select one. *What to do...*

- **Choose a multi made especially for women.** Women's multis typically provide extra folic acid, which protects against heart disease, colon cancer and birth defects...and extra bone-building calcium, magnesium and vitamin D.
- **Look for an age-appropriate formula.** Before menopause, it is common for monthly

blood loss to deplete the iron that red blood cells need—which is why women's multis often contain iron. Excess iron supplementation can damage organs, however—so if you're postmenopausal and have no diagnosed iron deficiency, it is wise to take an iron-free multi. Some "50+" formulas also provide extra B vitamins because the body's ability to absorb these often declines with age...and/or even higher amounts of calcium and vitamin D.

Good brands: Nature Made Multi for Her and Multi for Her 50+...One A Day Women's and Women's 50+ Advantage.

• **Supplement your supplement.** The daily value (DV)—the government-recommended daily intake—for calcium is 1,000 mg for women ages 19 to 50 and 1,200 mg for women over 50...the DV for magnesium is 400 mg. But many multis provide just a fraction of those DVs—otherwise, the pills would be too big.

Another problem: The DV for vitamin D is 400 international units (IU), an amount that many multis provide—yet experts advise getting 1,000 IU to 2,000 IU of vitamin D to lower risk for osteoporosis, diabetes, heart disease and some cancers.

Best: In addition to a multi, take a supplement that helps make up for these shortfalls, such as Caltrate 600-D Plus Minerals or Schiff Super Calcium-Magnesium...take additional vitamin D if necessary.

Clean Out Your Arteries

Mark A. Stengler, NMD, naturopathic medical doctor in private practice, Encinitas, California...adjunct associate clinical professor at the National College of Natural Medicine, Portland, Oregon...author of many books, including *The Natural Physician's Healing Therapies* and coauthor of *Prescription for Natural Cures* (both from Bottom Line Books)...and author of the *Bottom Line/ Natural Healing* newsletter.

Amid the clamor created by pharmaceutical companies hyping cholesterol-lowering statin drugs, important information is going unheard.

You need to know: Four natural therapies can protect, and even restore, the health of your arteries—without the dangerous side effects of statin drugs.

These natural substances help to reverse the process of plaque buildup—to dissolve plaque, eliminating the danger it presents. They are available over-the-counter from health-food stores, online and/or from holistic physicians. Unless otherwise noted, they have no serious side effects, can be taken indefinitely and are generally safe for everyone, including people who take statin drugs. *Important...*

• **If you have atherosclerosis or any other cardiovascular condition,** you need to be under a cardiologist's care.

• **If you take blood-thinning medication, such as aspirin or *warfarin* (Coumadin)—** typically given to improve blood flow and prevent blood clots—talk to your doctor before using the natural therapies below, because they could affect your medication dosage.

• **If you are pregnant,** speak to your doctor before taking these or any other supplements or drugs.

• **Discontinue use of these substances 10 to 14 days prior to scheduled surgery** to reduce the risk of excess bleeding. Resume use according to your doctor's instructions (typically 10 days after the procedure).

• **To determine which substance or combination of substances to use,** see "The Right Regimen for You" at the end of this article.

1. Tocotrienols. Vitamin E is not just one vitamin, but rather a family of eight slightly different molecular structures that function differently in the body. There are two principal categories of vitamin E, called *tocopherols* and *tocotrienols.* Each of these has four subcategories—alpha, beta, gamma and delta.

Some vitamin E supplements contain synthetic alpha-tocopherol. If that's what is in your cupboard—indicated on the label as "dl-alpha-tocopherol"—throw it out! Synthetic alpha-tocopherol hogs the space on cells' vitamin E receptors (slots into which molecules must fit in order to be used by the body), leaving less room for the more healthful tocopherols you ingest from food or from natural supplements (labeled "d-alpha-tocopherol"). Natural tocopherols reduce free radicals, helping to prevent new plaque, but they have not been shown to reduce plaque that is already present. For that, you need tocotrienols.

Tocotrienols are found in rice bran, coconut, barley and wheat germ—but only in small amounts. Supplements with mixed tocopherols/tocotrienols are sold in health-food stores—but they are not the best for reducing plaque.

Better: A tocotrienol-only supplement. I like Allergy Research Group Delta-Fraction Tocotrienols (800-545-9960, *www.allergyresearchgroup.com*), available from holistic doctors. The dosage is 300 milligrams (mg) per day.

2. Vitamin K. Vitamin K protects against harmful arterial calcification. Forms of vitamin K include *phylloquinone* (K-1) and *menaquinone* (K-2). Vitamin K-1 is abundant in dark green leafy vegetables, such as lettuce, spinach and broccoli. However, vitamin K-2 is better absorbed and remains active in the body longer than vitamin K-1. Good food sources of vitamin K-2 include natto (fermented soybeans) and, to a lesser degree, fermented cheeses (the type with holes, such as Swiss and Jarlsberg), beef liver, chicken and egg yolks.

People taking warfarin are at higher risk for atherosclerosis and osteoporosis (brittle bones) due to the drug's effects on calcification. A study in *Pharmacotherapy* demonstrated the safety and benefit of low-dose vitamin K supplementation in patients taking warfarin. Vitamin K also promotes beneficial bone calcification.

Note: It is vital that a person who takes blood thinners use vitamin K only under the close supervision of a doctor, because the medication dosage may need to be adjusted.

Research suggests that most people get too little vitamin K. I think daily supplementation with 150 to 200 micrograms (mcg) of vitamin K-2 is appropriate for all adults—and especially important for those with atherosclerosis. If you take warfarin, the daily dose may be modified, depending on blood tests that indicate how your clotting mechanism interacts with vitamin K. A brand I like is Jarrow Formula's MK-7 (310-204-6936, *www.jarrow.com*).

3. Garlic extract. Most beneficial is aged garlic extract (AGE), available in capsule or liquid form. A study from the University of California, Los Angeles, involved 19 cardiac patients who were taking statin drugs and aspirin daily. Participants took either a placebo or 4 milliliters (ml) of a liquid brand called Kyolic AGE for one year.

Findings: Participants who took AGE had about a 66% reduction in new plaque formation compared with those who took a placebo.

Research demonstrates that AGE also can...

- **Reduce LDL cholesterol by up to 12%... total cholesterol by up to 31%...and triglycerides by up to 19%.**
- **Protect against the LDL oxidation** that can trigger arterial plaque formation.
- **Thin the blood.**
- **Lower blood pressure.**
- **Reduce blood levels of homocysteine—** the amino acid that, when elevated, may raise cardiovascular disease risk.
- **Reduce C-reactive protein, which is a blood marker of inflammation and a risk factor for atherosclerosis.**
- **Combat carotid plaque.**

I recommend supplementing daily with AGE.

Dosage: 4 milliliters (ml) to 6 ml of liquid AGE or 400 mg to 600 mg in tablet or capsule form.

4. Pomegranate juice. Once considered exotic, pomegranate juice can now be found in supermarkets and is a proven boon to arterial health. Israeli researchers verified this in a three-year study of 19 men and women, ages 65 to 75, with severe carotid artery blockage. Ten participants drank 50 ml (two ounces) per day of 100% pomegranate juice, and nine participants drank a placebo.

Results: Among juice drinkers, plaque thickness decreased by an average of 13% after three months and 35% after one year. This is phenomenal—no drug can come close to reducing plaque like this! Placebo drinkers had a 9% increase in plaque after one year.

Pomegranate juice is loaded with antioxidants called *polyphenols*, which prevent cholesterol oxidation and improve blood flow.

Note: Choose 100% juice with no added sugar. Pomegranate juice contains a lot of naturally occurring sugar, so dilute two to four ounces of juice with an equal amount of water. Drink it with meals to slow the absorption of sugar into the bloodstream and help to maintain stable blood glucose levels. Use twice daily.

THE RIGHT REGIMEN FOR YOU

Arterial plaque buildup can be detected and its severity gauged using imaging tests, such as computed tomography (CT), magnetic resonance imaging (MRI) scan and/or ultrasound. Results help to determine the appropriate therapy for you. Tests may be repeated periodically to see if your regimen needs to be modified.

The four natural substances described in this article, used alone or in combination (following the dosage guidelines in the main article), can improve the health of your arteries. Here's how to tell which ones are right for you.

Note: If you take blood-thinning medication, talk to your doctor before using these substances.

If you do not have atherosclerosis, take one or more of these:

- **Vitamin K**
- **Aged garlic extract (AGE)**
- **Pomegranate juice**

For mild atherosclerosis, take all of these:

- **Vitamin K**
- **AGE**
- **Pomegranate juice**

For moderate or severe atherosclerosis, take all of these:

- **Tocotrienols**
- **Vitamin K**
- **AGE**
- **Pomegranate juice**
- **Statin medication**—but only if you and your doctor are not satisfied with your level of improvement after 12 months of daily use of all four natural substances.

Vitamin B-3 Beats Cholesterol Drug

Many cardiovascular disease patients who take cholesterol-lowering statins also take *ezetimibe* (Zetia) to combat cholesterol even further.

New study: Ezetimibe reduced LDL "bad" cholesterol but also reduced HDL "good" cholesterol and had no effect on artery wall thickness. In comparison, among patients who took 2 grams (g) daily of niacin (vitamin B-3) instead of Zetia, LDL dropped...HDL rose...arterial wall thickness was reduced (a desirable effect)...and there were significantly fewer adverse cardiac events.

Best: Ask your internist or cardiologist about how to use niacin safely since the various B vitamins are best taken in a balanced combination.

Allen J. Taylor, MD, director of advanced cardiovascular imaging, Washington Hospital Center, Washington, DC, and leader of a study of 208 cardiovascular patients.

Supplements vs. Drugs

Supplements beat cholesterol-lowering drugs. In a 12-week study of 74 adults who did not have heart disease but did have high LDL "bad" cholesterol levels (155 mg/dL, on average), one group took 40 mg daily of the statin drug *simvastatin* (Zocor). The other group took fish oil (three capsules daily) and red yeast rice supplements (2,400 mg to 3,600 mg daily) and made lifestyle changes, such as limiting fat intake and exercising five to six times weekly.

Result: LDL levels dropped by 42%, on average, in the supplement/lifestyle change group and 39%, on average, in the statin group. Talk to your doctor before trying such supplement/lifestyle therapy.

David J. Becker, MD, cardiologist, Chestnut Hill Hospital and the University of Pennsylvania Health System, both in Philadelphia.

Heart Supplements That Can Save Your Life

Dennis Goodman, MD, a clinical associate professor of medicine at New York University School of Medicine in New York City and at the University of California in San Diego. Dr. Goodman also is director of integrative medicine at New York Medical Associates, a group private practice in New York City. He is board certified in internal medicine, cardiology, interventional cardiology, critical care, clinical lipidology and holistic (integrative) medicine. *www.dennisgoodmanmd.com.*

One of the most common reasons that people take nutritional supplements is to improve their heart health.

Problem: Very few cardiologists are aware of the ways in which heart supplements work synergistically—that is, by taking carefully selected supplements in combinations, you will heighten the effectiveness of each one. Over the past 22 years, I have treated thousands of heart patients with this approach.

What you need to know to make the most of your nondrug regimen for better heart health...*

THE ESSENTIAL THREE

There are three daily supplements that I recommend to anyone who is concerned about heart health...

- **Fish oil capsules** primarily lower harmful blood fats known as triglycerides but also have a mild blood pressure–lowering effect.

Typical dose: 1 gram (g) total of the omega-3 fatty acids *eicosapentaenoic acid* (EPA) and *docosahexaenoic acid* (DHA) for blood pressure benefits. To reduce triglyceride levels, the typical daily dose is 2 g to 4 g total of EPA and DHA.

Caution: Fish oil can increase bleeding risk, so talk to your doctor if you take a blood thinner, such as *warfarin* (Coumadin).

- **CoQ10** helps enhance energy production in cells and inhibits blood clot formation.

Typical dose: 50 milligrams (mg) to 100 mg per day. CoQ10, which is commonly taken with the classic HDL-boosting treatment niacin (vitamin B-3), also helps minimize side effects, such as muscle weakness, in people taking cholesterol-lowering statin drugs.

- **Red yeast rice** is an extract of red yeast that is fermented on rice and is available in tablet, capsule, powder and liquid form. Long used by the Chinese, it mimics the action of cholesterol-lowering statin drugs.

Typical dose: 600 mg twice daily.

Red yeast rice is often used in combination with *plant sterols*, naturally occurring chemical compounds found in small amounts in fruits, vegetables and nuts...and added to food products, including butter substitutes, such as Promise activ and Benecol spreads.

Typical dose: About 400 mg daily of plant sterols.

Also important: Low levels of vitamin D (below 15 ng/mL) have been linked to a 62% increase, on average, in heart attack risk.

Typical dose: 5,000 international units (IU) of vitamin D-3 per day for those who are deficient in the vitamin...at least 1,000 IU daily for all other adults.

BETTER BLOOD PRESSURE CONTROL

The heart-friendly properties of fish oil are so well-documented that the American Heart Association endorses its use (by eating fatty fish at least twice weekly and/or taking fish oil capsules).

To enhance the blood pressure–lowering effect of fish oil, ask your doctor about adding...

- **L-arginine.** This amino acid boosts the body's production of the chemical compound nitric oxide, which causes the blood vessels to dilate, thereby lowering blood pressure.

Typical dose: 150 mg daily.

L-arginine is also used to treat erectile dysfunction and *claudication* (impeded blood flow in the extremities) and has a mild and beneficial HDL-boosting effect.

Caution: L-arginine should not be taken by children or pregnant or nursing women, or by anyone with genital herpes—it can stimulate activity of the herpes virus. Possible side effects include indigestion, nausea and headache.

- **Lycopene.** This phytochemical is found in tomatoes—especially processed tomato sauce—watermelon, pink grapefruit, red bell

*To find a doctor to oversee your heart-health supplement regimen, consult the American Board of Intergrative Holistic Medicine, *www.holisticboard.org.*

peppers and papaya. I usually recommend that patients try L-arginine first, then add lycopene, if necessary, for blood pressure reduction.

Research conducted at Ben-Gurion University in Israel has shown that lycopene lowers systolic (top number) blood pressure by up to 10 points and diastolic (bottom number) by up to four points.

A potent antioxidant, lycopene is also thought to have potential cancer-preventive effects, but this has not been proven.

Typical dose: 10 mg daily.

In rare cases, lycopene supplements can cause diarrhea and/or nausea. Because tomatoes and other acidic foods can aggrvate ulcer pain, people with stomach ulcers should consult their doctors before consuming tomatoes and tomato-based products regularly.

BOOST HDL CHOLESTEROL

In addition to taking CoQ10 and niacin, ask your doctor about trying...

- **Policosanol.** This plant-wax derivative has been found to boost HDL levels by more than 7%. The research on policosanol is considered controversial by some, but I have found it to be an effective HDL booster in my practice.

Typical dose: 10 mg daily.

There is also some evidence that policosanol may have LDL- and triglyceride-lowering benefits. There are no known side effects associated with policosanol.

Bonus: Used together, CoQ10, niacin and policosanol will allow you to raise your HDL levels while taking much lower doses of niacin (about 20 mg daily). A lower niacin dose reduces the risk for facial flushing, a common side effect in people who take the vitamin.

REDUCE LDL CHOLESTEROL

Red yeast rice extract and plant sterols (both described earlier) are well-known natural methods of lowering LDL cholesterol levels.

To lower your LDL cholesterol further, ask your doctor about adding policosanol (described earlier), along with...

- **Pantethine.** This is a more biologically active form of pantothenic acid (vitamin B-5).

Typical dose: 600 mg daily.

Numerous small studies have found that pantethine significantly lowers LDL cholesterol and triglycerides.

- **Grape seed extract.** This antioxidant-rich substance reduces the blood's tendency to clot and helps lower blood pressure by boosting levels of the chemical compound nitric oxide found in the body. Some research shows that grape seed extract reduces LDL cholesterol as well.

Typical dose: 200 mg daily.

In addition, studies suggest that grape seed extract may help protect against Alzheimer's disease.

Caution: Because grape seed extract has a blood-thinning effect, it should not be taken by anyone who uses warfarin or other blood-thinning medications or supplements.

Exciting New Health Benefits of CoQ10

Peter H. Langsjoen, MD, a cardiologist in private practice in Tyler, Texas, who specializes in noninvasive treatment. He is an active researcher and world-recognized expert in the biomedical benefits of CoQ10. A fellow of the American College of Cardiology, Dr. Langsjoen was a founding member of the International Coenzyme Q10 Association, *www.icqa.org.*

Until recently, the dietary supplement coenzyme Q10 (CoQ10) was recommended primarily for people who wanted to avoid the side effects of cholesterol-lowering statin drugs, including muscle pain and weakness.

Now: Researchers are discovering that CoQ10 may confer a variety of other health benefits that are unrelated to statin use.

Peter H. Langsjoen, MD,* is one of the world's foremost CoQ10 researchers. *He provided some background on the supplement and outlined the latest developments in the research...*

WHAT IS COQ10?

CoQ10 is a vitamin-like substance that plays a key role in the production of energy in every cell in the body. Discovered in 1957, the substance is naturally present in such foods as organ meats (including cow's liver and kidney), and, in smaller amounts, in beef, sardines, mackerel and peanuts. Because CoQ10 appeared to be everywhere in the body—or "ubiquitous"—it was dubbed *ubiquinone.*

Without adequate levels of CoQ10, the body's organs and systems, including the immune system and nervous system, will not function optimally.

UNEXPECTED HEALTH BENEFITS

Increasing scientific evidence now offers support for the use of CoQ10 supplements to help treat...

• **Heart disease.** CoQ10 is involved in creating 90% of cellular energy in the heart.

Research has shown that people with heart failure (inadequate pumping action of the heart) have lower blood levels of CoQ10, on average, than people without heart failure—and the lower the CoQ10 level, the worse the problem.

Recent research published in the journal *Biofactors* showed that the ejection fraction (the amount of blood pumped with each heartbeat) in heart failure patients who took CoQ10 supplements rose from an average of 22% to an average of 39% after six to 12 months.

Important: Because statin medications deplete the body's supply of CoQ10, ask your doctor about adding CoQ10 supplements (to help protect the heart and counteract statin-related side effects) to your regimen if you take one of these drugs.

• **High blood pressure.** CoQ10 can also help improve high blood pressure (hypertension). Studies have shown that about half of people using one or more drugs for high blood pressure can stop taking at least some of their medications after taking CoQ10 supplements for about five months.

• **Cholesterol.** CoQ10 also acts as a powerful antioxidant. It is transported in the blood (along with cholesterol and other fat-soluble nutrients) and helps protect cholesterol from damaging oxidation, which plays a role in atherosclerosis (fatty buildup in the arteries).

*Dr. Langsjoen has no financial interest in any company that manufactures or sells CoQ10 supplements.

• **Fatigue.** Because CoQ10 is part of the body's energy-producing processes, it is particularly valuable in reducing fatigue—even among people with severe fatigue, including that caused by such conditions as chronic fatigue syndrome.

• **Migraines.** In one study, 32 people who took CoQ10 supplements for three months had only half their usual number of migraines.

• **Neurological disorders.** Some of the most promising recent research involves the ability of CoQ10 to slow the progression of degenerative neurological disorders, including Parkinson's disease, Alzheimer's disease and Huntington's disease (a genetic disorder).

HOW TO USE COQ10 SAFELY

People who eat organ meats at least once or twice weekly usually have healthy CoQ10 levels. But other adults can improve their blood levels of CoQ10 by taking supplements. Work with your doctor to find an optimal dose.

For best absorption, do not take more than 180 milligrams (mg) at one time. CoQ10 is fat-soluble (dissolves in fat), so it is best to take the supplement with meals that contain at least a little bit of fat (any type).

In some people, CoQ10 may cause temporary side effects, such as nausea and other gastrointestinal disorders...dizziness...insomnia...or headache. However, these side effects are rare. If you experience side effects, try a different CoQ10 formulation.

Caution: One case study suggested that CoQ10 may act like vitamin K, lessening the blood-thinning effect of *warfarin* (Coumadin). But a controlled trial subsequently found no such effects.

Nevertheless, people taking warfarin or any other blood-thinning medication should consult a doctor before taking a CoQ10 supplement. After a few weeks of taking CoQ10, anyone who uses a blood thinner should have his/her *prothrombin time* (a measure of clotting ability) checked.

Also important: Because CoQ10 may cause your blood pressure and/or blood sugar (glucose) level to gradually improve, your doctor may want to adjust the dosage of any medications you may be taking to control elevations of either.

FINDING THE BEST PRODUCT

One reliable producer of CoQ10 is the Japanese company Kaneka, which sells CoQ10 in the US under many different brand names, including Healthy Origins (888-228-6650, *www.healthyorigins.com*) and Jarrow Formulas, available through ProVitaminas (800-510-6444, *www.provitaminas.com*). Kaneka uses a yeast fermentation process with 99.9% pure natural CoQ10.

In addition to CoQ10 supplements, you may see products labeled "ubiquinol." Ubiquinol is a more bioavailable (absorbable)—and more expensive—form of CoQ10. However, if you take CoQ10, your body will naturally convert it to ubiquinol. While most healthy adults readily absorb CoQ10, patients with advanced heart failure absorb ubiquinol about four times better than CoQ10.

If you purchase ubiquinol (not CoQ10), test it for freshness (in case it has deteriorated during storage or shipping).

What to do: Cut a capsule in half, and look at the color of the contents. Cream-colored is good—orange or brown means that the product has become oxidized.

Whichever form you choose, shop around—a month's supply of a high-quality supplement can cost $20 to about $60.

Fish Oil

Mark A. Stengler, NMD, naturopathic medical doctor in private practice, Encinitas, California...adjunct associate clinical professor at the National College of Natural Medicine, Portland, Oregon...author of many books, including *The Natural Physician's Healing Therapies* and coauthor of *Prescription for Natural Cures* (both from Bottom Line Books)...and author of the *Bottom Line/Natural Healing* newsletter.

Among the essential fatty acids that we need to live, omega-3s are very important. These are fats that your body can't manufacture on its own, so they need to come from food sources or supplements.

While omega-3 is also found in flaxseed and flaxseed oil, the kind that you get from fish and fish oil has some unique properties that are not present in these other foods. The fish and fish oils are a direct source of two long-chain fatty acids known as EPA (*eicosapentanoic acid*) and DHA (*docosahexanoic acid*), and both are very important for heart health.

Another reason doctors are confident about the benefits of fish oil is pragmatic. The vast majority of studies on essential fatty acids have been done on fish oils. There are sound reasons to believe that oils such as flaxseed oil may be nearly as effective, but to date, they haven't been studied so much. It is the fish oils that have been studied and shown to be effective.

Fish became more popular as a "healthy heart" food when researchers studied the "Mediterranean diet"—that is, the diet of many cultures around the Mediterranean during the 1960s in Crete, parts of Greece, and southern Italy. (There, as in many other cultures, the "American diet" has crept in, raising the rate of heart disease and other chronic diseases). In the classic Mediterranean diet, people had many plant foods (vegetables, legumes, fruit, bread, pasta, nuts), lots of olive oil, and low to moderate amounts of fish, poultry, meat, dairy, eggs, and wine.

Nutritionists believe the consumption of fish was one of the key benefits of this diet, which resulted in a much lower incidence of obesity, heart disease, diabetes, and cancer. A four-year study of the Mediterranean diet found that people could reduce their risk of heart attack by as much as 70 percent.

SEA RATIONS

In a more direct study of fish consumption, a team of researchers who looked at mortality data from 36 countries confirmed that life expectancy is longer in those countries where people get a lot of fish in their daily diet. Men and women who eat more fish have a lower risk of early death from all kinds of illnesses, particularly stroke and heart disease.

Essential fatty acids form a group of hormone-like messengers known as prostaglandins. The omega-3 fatty acids as found in fish oil—helped along by the EPA and DHA in the fish—tend to decrease inflammation, thin the blood, and balance the immune system.

In the immune system, EPA appears to be particularly important for its antiinflammatory effects, so it's helpful to people who have arthritis. DHA is critical for the proper development and function of the brain because your brain cells need it to transmit electrical impulses efficiently. It's not surprising, therefore, that a DHA deficiency can lead to memory, behavior, and learning problems.

Some studies have also indicated that supplementing infant formula with DHA can improve children's IQ. Interestingly, it's also important for mood regulation, and studies have shown that a deficiency can contribute to depression.

The DHA found in fish oil also appears to calm down hyperactive children. It is also required for proper retinal development for infants.

DOSAGE

Fish oil capsules generally are available in 500- to 1,000-milligram doses. When purchasing the capsules, pay particular attention to the amounts of EPA and DHA stated on the labels. You want fish oils that contain about 18 percent EPA and 12 percent DHA: in other words, totalling about 30 percent of the omega-3 fatty acids found in these fish oils. (Some of the newly developed, high-potency fish oils now contain even higher concentrations of EPA and DHA.)

For preventative purposes, I recommend that people eat foods high in DHA and EPA such as cold-water fish. (Eggs also contain DHA.)

If your health is generally good, I'd advise taking 2,000 milligrams (mg) of a daily fish-oil supplement such as salmon oil. But if you're susceptible to specific diseases such as arthritis, high blood pressure, and other conditions, I'd advise getting a higher dose—as much as 6,000 to 10,000 milligrams per day. However, you'll probably want to check with your health practitioner to find an optimal dose for your condition, since the supplement can be costly.

If you're taking the concentrated fish-oil capsules that have higher concentrations of EPA and DHA, I recommend salmon oil or tuna oil capsules that have been tested for heavy metal contamination and rancidity. I am also a big fan of the oil blends that contain a combination of essential fatty acids such as DHA, EPA, and GLA. An ideal formula also has vitamin E in it. If not, take vitamin E with the fish oil to prevent the oil from going rancid.

Fish-oil capsules should be stored in the refrigerator once they are opened. Don't leave the container standing in bright light or keep it in a warm room.

WHAT ARE THE SIDE EFFECTS?

Some people who take fish oil experience digestive upset including burping—which can be disconcerting because you may burp a "fishy" smell. But you probably won't have that problem if you take the capsules with meals.

Since fish oils also have a blood-thinning effect, check with your doctor if you are taking any blood-thinning medications.

You may have an increase in LDL cholesterol while supplementing fish oil. If a blood test shows your cholesterol count is on the rise, you can take a garlic supplement to help neutralize this potential effect of the fish oil.

Although people have relatively few and minor problems with the side effects of fish oil, there's a risk that the capsules can contain rancid oil. It's easy to check, however. Just cut open the end of a capsule. If the fish oil has gone rancid, you can easily smell the strong odor. You're better off getting a fresh bottle with new capsules.

Finally, check the label of any brand you buy to make sure the product was tested for contaminants such as heavy metals.

FISH OIL

My recommendations for...

• ADD and ADHD

Many school-age children have been diagnosed with attention deficit disorder (ADD) or attention deficit hyperactivity disorder (ADHD), and their problems are sometimes related to nutritional imbalances. (Excess sugars and some additives in junk food have particularly been blamed.)

Essential fatty acids such as DHA are critically important for proper brain function, but—well, how many children do you know who eat fresh cold-water fish three times a week? When children aren't getting enough

DHA and they're loading up on saturated fat, trans fatty acids, and omega-6 fatty acids from fast-foods, the inevitable result is a fatty-acid imbalance.

• Arthritis

Numerous studies with fish oil have been done on people with rheumatoid arthritis and the results have been very positive. For aggressive treatment using fish oil, take 6,000 milligrams daily. Some people need doses that are even higher, so talk to your health practitioner about the optimum dose if you have severe rheumatoid arthritis.

If the fish oil is helpful in reducing stiffness and pain, there's a good chance you'll be able to reduce the dosages of pharmaceuticals. Drug therapy for rheumatoid arthritis focuses on *prednisone*, *methotrexate* (also used for chemotherapy), and anti-inflammatory medications—all of which can have serious toxicity when used on a long-term basis. With fish oil, on the other hand, there's no toxicity, so it's a far more benign treatment than the classic pharmaceuticals. One study found that many patients were able to go off their anti-inflammatory drugs while supplementing fish oil and experienced no relapse in their rheumatoid arthritis. Researchers found that the fish oil had a balancing effect on the entire immune system.

It is recommended, as the result of studies, that a minimum daily dose of 3,000 milligrams EPA and DHA is necessary to derive the expected benefits, although I find not all my patients need this high a dosage. Once you start taking fish oil, you can expect to stay on it for at least 12 weeks before it begins to yield benefits. But after that, you can stay on it indefinitely.

• Asthma

The rate of asthma keeps increasing. Sadly, children's asthma is continuing to rise at an alarming rate. Environmental pollution and poor dietary habits are largely to blame.

Essential fatty acids in fish and fish oil help to suppress the inflammatory chemicals involved in this disease. Studies show that children who eat oily fish more than once a week have one-third the risk of getting asthma as children who do not eat fish or eat lean fish on a regular basis.

Fish-oil supplements are helpful for both children and adults with asthma. Again, the benefits of fish oil take months before the natural anti-inflammatory benefits begin to take hold.

• Cancer

Omega-3 fatty acids are important for a healthy, well-functioning immune system. If you can get more omega-3 fatty acids in your diet and also take supplements, there's a good chance you can help protect yourself from certain types of cancers.

Animal studies have shown that fish oil can augment certain types of chemotherapy to fight cancer more effectively. Fish oil has also been shown to help treat cachexia, which is the loss of muscle mass and weight in cancer patients.

• Cardiovascular Disease

With many studies to back up its benefits, fish oil is often recommended as a preventative for heart and circulation problems. Along with the population studies showing that consumption of fish oil slashes the rate of cardiovascular disease, are literally hundreds of studies that support these observations. Fish oils reduce cholesterol and triglyceride levels and also act as a natural blood thinner, which results in the lowering of blood pressure.

• Chronic Obstructive Pulmonary Disease

Over 17 million Americans suffer from this group of serious breathing disorders that includes asthma, bronchitis, and emphysema. Smoking, as you might expect, is the factor that multiplies your chances of getting any of these diseases. But for smokers as well as nonsmokers, there are some benefits in eating fish as often as possible.

• Crohn's Disease and Ulcerative Colitis

Inflammatory bowel diseases such as Crohn's disease and ulcerative colitis can be helped by fish-oil supplementation.

In one study of ulcerative colitis, people who took fish-oil supplements (high in omega-3s) were able to cut their steroid medications in half. Again, I see fish oil as one component of a total natural-therapy program to address and alleviate these digestive conditions. Other measures include stress reduction, improving digestive capacity, and maintaining a healthful diet.

Herbal medicines and homeopathy are excellent therapies to help turn these conditions around without relying on pharmaceutical drugs that may have many damaging side effects.

• Depression

The brain is 60 percent fat and requires essential fatty acids, especially DHA, to function properly. It has been shown that people deficient in DHA are much more likely to suffer from depression.

Consuming fish on a regular basis is a good way to prevent depression. I recommend concentrated DHA supplements for those already battling depression.

• Eczema

I have found that flaxseeds and flaxseed oil in combination with GLA work well for eczema. It also makes sense to consume cold-water fish rich in omega-3 fatty acids. Fish oil is also another option to treat eczema.

• High Blood Pressure

High blood pressure is one of the biggest risk factors for heart disease and stroke. Numerous studies have shown that fish oil reduces blood pressure. I find fish oil works best as part of a natural program—combined with stress-reduction techniques and a regimen that includes herbs such as hawthorn, minerals such as magnesium and calcium, along with the natural supplement CoQ10.

• High Triglycerides

With fish oil, you can lower high triglyceride levels, which are an independent risk factor for heart disease. As I've mentioned, though, fish oil can increase LDL cholesterol, so you'll want to supplement with garlic to help balance out its effects.

• Insulin Resistance

The inability to metabolize carbohydrates effectively leads to high blood-sugar levels and a corresponding spike of the hormone insulin (the component that helps get the blood sugar into the cells). As a result, many different biochemical reactions can occur, one of which is weight gain.

Clinical studies have shown that omega-3 fatty acids, such as those in fish oil, help improve the body's utilization of insulin. (It's interesting that an essential fatty acid can help decrease body fat!) This insulin-balancing effect is also important in relation to diabetes.

• Kidney Protection

People who receive organ transplants require extensive immune-suppressing drugs. These are needed to keep the body from rejecting the donated organ, but some of the drugs (such as *cyclosporine*) are so powerful that they can have life-threatening side effects.

In the case of patients who have had kidney transplants, however, it's been shown that they resume normal kidney function more quickly when omega-3–rich fish oil is supplemented. It appears that the fish oil actually protects the kidneys from the damaging effects of the immune-suppressing drugs.

• Lupus

Two pilot studies have shown fish oil to benefit people with lupus, an autoimmune condition where the immune system attacks its own tissue. For patients with lupus, I suggest eating cold-water fish regularly and supplementing with fish oil. It may take six months to a year before there's any improvement, but sometimes the benefits can be dramatic.

• Multiple Sclerosis

Dr. Roy Swank, the doctor who developed a natural protocol for multiple sclerosis (MS), recommended fish oil as well as flaxseed oil. In fact, Dr. Swank advocated that patients who have MS should eat fish three times a week or more. He was also a proponent of cod liver oil—one of the popular fish oils—as a daily supplement.

• Psoriasis

Several studies have shown that 10 to 12 grams of fish oil daily can improve psoriasis. I routinely recommend fish oil and dietary fish as well as other natural therapies to improve this inflammatory condition.

• Schizophrenia

Some preliminary studies are showing that EPA and DHA may be helpful in the treatment of schizophrenia. More research needs to be done, but I would not be surprised to see these essential fatty acids become accepted as part of the routine treatment for schizophrenia. Dr. Abraham Hoffer of Victoria, Canada has already demonstrated that a knowledgeable practitioner can provide a full-scale treatment of schizophrenia with nutritional therapies.

The Simple Supplement That May Prevent Killer Diseases

Joseph Maroon, MD, a professor of neurological surgery and Heindl Scholar in Neuroscience at the University of Pittsburgh School of Medicine and team neurosurgeon for the Pittsburgh Steelers. He is the author of *The Longevity Factor: How Resveratrol and Red Wine Activate Genes for a Longer and Healthier Life* (Atria). *www.josephmaroon.com.*

When it comes to "hot" supplements, *resveratrol* is high on the list. Multiple studies conducted on laboratory animals have demonstrated the highly beneficial effects of this *polyphenol* (a class of plant chemicals), which is found most abundantly in the skins of grapes and in red wine—and now is available in supplement form.

Key animal findings: Resveratrol has been shown not only to enhance muscle strength and reduce fatigue, but also to help prevent heart disease, stroke, diabetes and cancer...clear away the toxic proteins that cause Alzheimer's disease...and even lengthen life span by 25%.

But can this substance accomplish the same for humans?

AN IMPORTANT DISCOVERY

Resveratrol's emergence as an anti-aging and disease-fighting powerhouse began in the 1930s with a seemingly unrelated finding—that severe calorie restriction extended the lives of rodents by 40% to 50%.

It wasn't until the 1990s, however, that researchers at Harvard Medical School discovered the genetic basis for the beneficial effect of calorie restriction. Through various experiments in animal studies, calorie restriction was shown to trigger a kind of chain reaction that activates "survival genes" (*sirtuins*), which, in turn, energize an enzyme (SIR2) that stabilizes DNA. This process slows cellular aging. In further studies, researchers discovered that resveratrol is one of the most potent sources of the molecules that activate these survival genes.

CURRENT EVIDENCE

To further test resveratrol's benefits, researchers conducted other animal studies—this time without calorie restriction. Resveratrol and other polyphenols were found to increase the life span of fish by 60%...worms and flies by 30%...and mice by 25%—benefits attributed to improved cellular health.

Resveratrol-enhanced cells are believed to help fight...

- **Heart disease and stroke.** Resveratrol appears to decrease harmful inflammation, which contributes to cardiovascular disease.

Breakthrough research: A human study showed that drinking one-and-a-half glasses of red wine a day lowered, by 40%, levels of *lipid peroxide*, a by-product of inflammation that damages arteries. This and other health benefits are believed to be due to resveratrol and several other polyphenols in red wine.

Through various animal studies, resveratrol was shown to spark the production of the beneficial gas *nitric oxide*, which gives blood vessels more flexibility. Resveratrol also thins the blood, reducing the risk for a clot that will clog an artery. In studies of animals with induced heart attacks, those given resveratrol had a significantly lower fatality rate. In similar studies on stroke, resveratrol prevented paralysis and limited brain injury in animals.

- **Cancer.** Eighteen different types of cancer—including lung, colon, skin, liver and pancreatic—have been markedly inhibited by resveratrol in laboratory studies using both animal and human cells.

- **Diabetes.** In animals, resveratrol helps normalize blood sugar (glucose) levels by moving glucose out of the bloodstream and into cells. Laboratory research also shows that resveratrol reduces diabetic neuropathy (nerve pain that often occurs in the legs and feet).

Recent finding: In a human study, a synthetic, resveratrol-like compound was shown to give people the same type of glucose control that resveratrol gives mice.

• **Alzheimer's disease.** In animal studies, resveratrol helps remove the *amyloid-beta protein* that has been associated with Alzheimer's disease.

Recent finding: In a study of 90 healthy people, researchers at Marywood University in Scranton found that a supplement containing resveratrol and other polyphenols improved memory and sped up reaction time.

RESVERATROL SOURCES

Even though the preliminary research is promising, there is a caveat. You would have to drink up to 1,150 bottles of red wine daily to get the amount of resveratrol used in most animal studies.

Since that's not feasible, I recommend a more practical approach that includes two things—a regular diet of resveratrol- and polyphenol-rich foods (the resveratrol is far lower than the doses used in animal studies, but these foods contain other beneficial compounds that may enhance absorption of resveratrol from food and/or supplements)...and the use of a mixed polyphenol supplement or a resveratrol-only supplement.

That strategy—along with exercise and a lifestyle that includes the health-promoting effects of close emotional ties with family and friends—is your best bet for fighting chronic disease and living longer. *My advice...*

• **Eat a polyphenol-rich diet.** Resveratrol is the superstar of polyphenols, but many scientists think that a combination of polyphenols—ingesting them together, as they are found in nature—is the best way to activate survival genes.

The foods richest in resveratrol and a variety of other polyphenols...

• **Red wine or red grape juice.** These are the top dietary sources of resveratrol.

Important: Wine grapes with the most resveratrol include pinot noir, merlot, grenache, cabernet sauvignon and tempranillo. (These wines also deliver up to about 500 different polyphenols along with resveratrol.)

Suggested daily intake: Four to 16 ounces of red grape juice daily (be mindful of the sugar content). Up to 12 ounces of red wine daily for men...and no more than six ounces daily for women (the potential health benefit of daily wine consumption by women must be weighed against a possible increase in breast cancer risk).

• **Pomegranate juice.** It is a good source of resveratrol and many other antioxidants.

Suggested daily intake: Three to five ounces.

• **Dark chocolate.** It is a rich source of concentrated *flavonols*, a potent type of polyphenol. Select unsweetened or semisweetened varieties with at least 70% cocoa. Suggested daily intake: One bite-sized square.

• **Green tea.** Green tea contains resveratrol and is rich in *epigallocatechin gallate* (EGCG) and other polyphenols. Suggested daily intake: Three eight-ounce cups. Decaffeinated green tea contains EGCG but relatively little resveratrol.

• **Blueberries.** They are rich in *procyanidins* and other polyphenols. Suggested daily intake: At least one cup (fresh or frozen).

• **Take a mixed-polyphenol supplement.** I recommend the mixed polyphenol supplement Vindure 900, a product developed by Vinomis Laboratories based on Harvard University research. Vindure is available from Vinomis Laboratories (877-484-6664, *www.vinomis.com*).

Because resveratrol absorption is thought to be enhanced when combined with other natural polyphenols, a mixed-polyphenol supplement is best.

However, an alternative is to...

• **Take a resveratrol supplement.** There are more than 300 resveratrol-containing products now available. The best products are made with *trans-resveratrol* (the active form of the substance shown by professional testing to activate the sirtuin "survival genes")...and produced by manufacturers who comply with "Good Manufacturing Practices" (GMP), which ensures that the product contains no major contaminants.

My favorite resveratrol products are manufactured by...

• **Longevinex,** *www.longevinex.com*, 866-405-4000.

• **RevGenetics,** at *www.revgenetics.com*, 888-738-4363.

Suggested intake for most resveratrol supplements: 250 mg to 500 mg daily.

Vitamin K: The Forgotten Vitamin

Sarah Booth, PhD, director of the Vitamin K Laboratory at the Jean Mayer USDA Human Nutrition and Research Center on Aging and a professor at the Gerald J. and Dorothy R. Friedman School of Nutrition Science and Policy, both at Tufts University in Boston. Dr. Booth has led or participated in more than 50 scientific studies on vitamin K.

Vitamin K is the first nutritional supplement that most Americans ever receive. That's because newborns routinely get a shot of the nutrient—which is crucial for coagulation (blood clotting)—to help prevent a severe and sometimes fatal bleeding disorder.

Discovered by a Danish scientist in 1934, the vitamin was dubbed "K" for "Koagulation" (the Danish spelling). But it wasn't until years later that scientists figured out how it works—by helping the liver manufacture several proteins that control blood clotting.

Latest development: Researchers are now discovering that vitamin K provides a wide variety of health benefits that extend well beyond blood clotting.

VITAMIN K FOR BETTER HEALTH

Vitamins C and E tend to get the most media attention, but recent findings on vitamin K's ability to help curb the development and/or progression of certain common medical ailments are worth noting.

Examples...

- **Arthritis.** Research shows that low dietary intake of vitamin K may play a role in the development of osteoarthritis.

Scientific evidence: In a study published in the journal *Arthritis & Rheumatism*, higher blood levels of dietary vitamin K were associated with a lower risk for osteoarthritis of the hand and knee.

- **Heart disease.** Vitamin K aids the function of the biochemical matrix *Gla-protein*, which helps prevent calcium buildup in plaque-filled arteries.

Scientific evidence: Researchers in the Netherlands studied more than 4,800 people over age 55. Compared with those with the lowest intake of vitamin K, those with the highest intake were 52% less likely to have severe calcification of the aorta, the major artery leading from the heart. The participants were 57% less likely to die of heart disease.

- **Liver cancer.** Cirrhosis of the liver, which occurs when alcoholism or infection with the hepatitis B or C virus results in scarred, abnormal liver tissue, can lead to liver cancer.

Scientific evidence: Studies of animal and human cells show that vitamin K may help control the progression of liver cancer. For example, in a study published in *The Journal of the American Medical Association*, Japanese researchers divided 40 women with viral cirrhosis of the liver into two groups. One group received vitamin K daily...the other did not. Two of the women in the vitamin K group developed liver cancer, compared with nine in the non-vitamin K group. Statistically, vitamin K lowered the risk for liver cancer by 80%.

- **Osteoporosis.** Vitamin K aids in the formation of *osteocalcin* (a protein that helps calcium bind to bone). This bone-strengthening process may help prevent and/or treat osteoporosis, the brittle-bone disease that afflicts more than 10 million older Americans—80% of them women.

Scientific evidence: Scientists at Harvard Medical School analyzed data on vitamin K intake and bone health in more than 70,000 women. Those with the highest dietary intake of vitamin K had a 30% decreased risk for hip fracture compared with those who had the lowest intake. Other studies show similar results for men.

In England, researchers analyzed data from 13 Japanese clinical trials that used large, pharmacological doses of vitamin K to treat osteoporosis. Overall, the vitamin reduced the rate of spinal fractures by 40% and hip fractures by 13%.

Latest development: Scientists at the University of Toronto, Tufts University and the University of Wisconsin have completed three clinical trials to determine whether nutritional doses of vitamin K can prevent bone loss in postmenopausal women. It is likely that researchers will present or publish their results within 12 months.*

ARE YOU GETTING ENOUGH?

The US government's recommended daily intake for vitamin K is 90 micrograms (mcg) for adult women...and 120 mcg for adult men. That level is high enough to prevent vitamin K deficiency, a rare condition that can lead to impaired blood clotting.

But is it high enough to keep your blood, bones and heart healthy? That's a question nutritional scientists are asking—but haven't yet answered.

However, scientists do know an easy, natural way to maximize your intake of vitamin K. It comes down to the classic maternal advice—eat your vegetables.

Green vegetables—leafy and otherwise—are among the best dietary sources of vitamin K. (For amounts, see box in adjacent column.)

Don't have a taste for kale or spinach? Don't worry. One-half cup of broccoli sautéed in olive oil gives you plenty of vitamin K. Or try a lettuce salad (using any type except iceberg) with a teaspoon of salad dressing that contains vegetable oil (some fat is needed for absorption of vitamin K). And don't worry about cooking—it doesn't destroy the vitamin.

Among vegetable oils, the richest sources of vitamin K (per two-tablespoon serving) are soybean oil (50 mcg) and olive oil (13 mcg).

Another good source: Mayonnaise (23 mcg).

Should you take a vitamin K supplement? Scientists don't have enough data at this point to recommend a dietary supplement of this nutrient for healthy adults.

IF YOU TAKE WARFARIN

Warfarin (Coumadin and Jantoven) is a widely used blood-thinning medication given to people who have had or are likely to develop an artery-blocking blood clot. Warfarin is often prescribed following a heart attack, stroke, blood clot in the leg (deep vein thrombosis) or a clot that has traveled to the lung (pulmonary embolism). The drug is also used in people who have an irregular heart rhythm (atrial fibrillation) or an artificial heart valve.

Warfarin works by decreasing the activity of vitamin K.

If you take warfarin: Don't eat dark, leafy green vegetables. The amount of vitamin K in these foods can vary threefold, depending on where they're grown. For example, a serving of spinach could contain 200 mcg of vitamin K...or 600 mcg. That's a significant difference in vitamin K intake for someone taking warfarin, who should not have large fluctuations in intake of this vitamin.

Instead, eat three daily servings of vitamin K–rich foods with lower but predictable amounts of the nutrient. That could include one-half cup of broccoli, one-half cup of green peas or six ounces of tomato juice. Other good choices of foods that contain relatively low amounts of vitamin K include asparagus and green beans.

To help determine the dose of warfarin that prevents blood cots from forming, doctors test the coagulation time—a measurement known as the International Normalized Ratio and Prothrombin Time (INR/PT). INR/PT is checked monthly, and the patient is instructed to maintain a consistent dietary intake of vitamin K to avoid altering the effectiveness of warfarin.

VITAMIN K IN VEGETABLES
(Estimated micrograms, per one-half cup, cooked)

	mcg
Kale	530
Collard greens	500
Spinach	440
Beet greens	350
Swiss chard	290
Turnip greens	260
Brussels sprouts	190
Dandelion greens	100
Broccoli	75
Asparagus	45
Cabbage	36
Green peas	20
Green beans	10

Source: US Department of Agriculture

*To stay abreast of this research, go to the National Institutes of Health Web site, *www.clinicaltrials.gov.*

Foods and Supplements That Prevent Cancer

Mark A. Stengler, NMD, naturopathic medical doctor in private practice, Encinitas, California...adjunct associate clinical professor at the National College of Natural Medicine, Portland, Oregon...author of many books, including *The Natural Physician's Healing Therapies* and coauthor of *Prescription for Natural Cures* (both from Bottom Line Books)...and author of the *Bottom Line/ Natural Healing* newsletter.

If you are confused about whether certain vitamins, supplements or foods can prevent cancer, you're not alone. The results of several recent studies have been conflicting and perplexing—which is why this topic has raised questions for consumers as well as members of the health-care and research communities.

What you need to know: Cancer is not a single disease, and it can have many different causes. That makes it virtually impossible for any one nutrient to protect against all types of cancer. In fact, studying whether single nutrients reduce the risk for cancer often is like looking for a magic bullet—more wishful thinking than good science.

Nothing can absolutely guarantee that you'll remain cancer free. However, good nutrition and a healthful overall lifestyle—not smoking, not abusing alcohol, limiting exposure to pollutants, eliminating food additives, exercising and controlling stress—can lower your odds of developing cancer. Here are my top five foods and top five supplements that definitely can lower your long-term risk of getting cancer.

MY TOP ANTICANCER FOODS

Consume a diet that emphasizes a variety of fresh, natural and minimally processed foods. Include a selection of vegetables, some fruits (such as berries and kiwifruit), fish, chicken (free-range or organic), legumes, nuts and modest amounts of healthful starches (such as sweet potatoes and whole grains). Eat healthfully—and you will lay the foundation for everything else that you can do to lower your long-term risk for cancer.

My favorite anticancer foods...

- **Broccoli.** Cruciferous vegetables are my top anticancer food, and broccoli heads the list. It is rich in *sulforaphane*, an antioxidant that helps the liver break down and destroy cancer-causing toxins. Sulforaphane also increases the activity of liver enzymes that help to get cancerous substances out of the body. (Sulforaphane is available as a supplement, although I recommend people get this phytonutrient through food.) Even better, broccoli sprouts contain 50 times more sulforaphane than that found in regular broccoli. A product called BroccoSprouts is available at select supermarkets (877-747-1277, *www.broccosprouts.com*). Broccoli sprouts also have been shown to fight *H. pylori*, a type of bacteria believed to cause stomach cancer.

Advice: Eat one-half cup of raw or lightly steamed broccoli daily. (Boiling reduces its nutritional value.) Add some broccoli sprouts to your salads or sandwiches.

- **Tomatoes.** This fruit is rich in lycopene, the antioxidant that gives tomatoes their red color. Studies have found that tomatoes reduce the risk for prostate cancer—and also might reduce the risk for lung and stomach cancers.

Advice: Consume cooked tomatoes or tomato sauce. Lycopene is best absorbed from cooked tomatoes because cooking breaks down the fiber in the tomatoes. A little fat (e.g., olive oil) also enhances absorption. Include one serving of tomato sauce (one-half cup) in your diet several times a week. Watermelon and guava also contain a lot of lycopene.

- **Cold-water fish.** Salmon, sardines and trout are rich in healthy omega-3 fats—specifically *eicosapentaenoic acid* (EPA) and *docosahexaenoic acid* (DHA). EPA and DHA have potent anti-inflammatory benefits. Low intake of these fats appears to be a factor in breast, colon, pancreatic and stomach cancers.

Advice: Eat cold-water fish at least once or twice a week, or take a fish oil supplement daily that contains 1 gram of EPA and DHA. Or use krill oil, a type of fish oil from shrimp-like crustaceans.

- **Garlic.** Slice or dice a garlic clove, and a relatively inert compound called *allicin* undergoes an amazing cascade of chemical changes.

Nearly all allicin-generated compounds function as antioxidants that prevent the types of cell mutations that give rise to cancer. Evidence suggests that garlic might help protect against cancers of the colon, prostate, esophagus, larynx, ovaries and kidneys.

Advice: Consume garlic regularly. Because chopping and cooking garlic seem to increase its biological activity, sauté or bake it rather than eating it whole or raw. There is no recommended serving size for garlic, but the more you consume, the better.

• **Spinach.** Spinach and other "greens," such as chard and collard greens, are rich in antioxidants that protect cells from the type of damage that can create cancerous mutations. One study published in *Journal of Agricultural and Food Chemistry* gave spinach the top "bioactivity index" ranking of vegetables for its ability to protect against cancer.

Advice: Eat spinach and other greens daily. You can make spinach salads or 50/50 lettuce and spinach salads, or gently sauté spinach. A single serving is equivalent to one cup of raw or one-half cup of cooked spinach or greens.

MY TOP ANTICANCER SUPPLEMENTS

Research on the role of individual supplements in reducing cancer risk has been especially confusing. *Taking all evidence into account, I'm convinced that these five supplements have clear benefits...*

• **Vitamin D.** If you were to take just one immune-enhancing supplement to lower your long-term risk for cancer, vitamin D would be the one to choose. More than 60 studies have found that high levels of vitamin D offer broad protection against many types of cancer. A recent German study reported that people with low vitamin D levels were one-third more likely to die of any type of cancer.

Advice: Take at least 1,000 international units (IU) of vitamin D-3 daily. Vitamin D-3, with its slightly different molecular structure than D-2, is a more bioactive form of the vitamin, which means that the body can use it more readily. Take 2,000 IU if you don't get much sun or have a dark complexion. (Dark skin absorbs less of the rays necessary for conversion to vitamin D.)

Best: Have your blood tested to determine how much vitamin D you need.

• **Vitamin K.** Two recent studies have shown an unexpected benefit of vitamin K—that it reduces the odds of developing breast and liver cancers.

Possible mechanism: Vitamin K activates *osteocalcin*, a protein involved in making strong bones. Recent research found that osteocalcin also may function as an anticancer nutrient.

Advice: Take 300 micrograms (mcg) of either vitamin K-1 or vitamin K-2, the forms most often studied.

Caution: Vitamin K may increase blood clotting. Do not take vitamin K if you also are taking blood-thinning medication unless you are being monitored by a doctor.

• **Selenium.** This essential dietary mineral forms part of *glutathione peroxidase*, an antioxidant enzyme that helps the liver break down cancer-causing toxins. A study published in *The Journal of the American Medical Association* found that 200 mcg daily of selenium led to significant reductions in the risk for prostate, colon and lung cancers within just a few years.

Advice: Take 200 mcg daily. Don't take a higher dose (which could be toxic) without the supervision of a nutrition-oriented doctor.

• **Coenzyme Q10 (CoQ10).** I believe that modest amounts of this vitamin-like nutrient may reduce an individual's general risk for cancer. Studies have shown that large amounts of CoQ10 can inhibit the spread of breast cancer and boost immunity...and may have benefits in other types of cancer as well. A recent study of women with breast cancer who were on the drug tamoxifen found that a combination of 100 milligrams (mg) of CoQ10 daily and vitamins B-2 (10 mg) and B-3 (50 mg) boosted the activity of enzymes that can repair genes.

Advice: Take 100 mg daily. If you already have been treated for cancer, take 300 mg daily.

• **Lycopene.** This antioxidant helps prevent cell damage. Several small studies have shown that lycopene supplements can reduce the size of prostate tumors and their tendency to spread. They also can lower levels of *prostate-specific antigen* (PSA), a common marker of prostate cancer risk.

Advice: For prostate cancer prevention and for men with elevated PSA levels, I recommend taking 5 mg to 10 mg of lycopene daily, even if you eat lycopene-rich foods. If you have been diagnosed with prostate cancer, discuss taking 30 mg daily with your physician. Use tomato-based (not synthetic) lycopene, which contains other beneficial antioxidants.

Note: Some multivitamins may contain these nutrients but not in the amounts recommended for cancer prevention. Check the label of your multivitamin, and add to it, based on the recommendations above.

Synthetic Vitamins

Mark A. Stengler, NMD, naturopathic medical doctor in private practice, Encinitas, California...adjunct associate clinical professor at the National College of Natural Medicine, Portland, Oregon...author of many books, including *The Natural Physician's Healing Therapies* and coauthor of *Prescription for Natural Cures* (both from Bottom Line Books)...and author of the *Bottom Line/Natural Healing* newsletter.

Many supplements that are marketed as "whole food blends" or "natural" have just the smallest amount of whole food or food extract. Adding whole foods to the mix does not magically make the nutrients "natural." Beware of these supplements—many are not worth the cost. Some supplements do contain some naturally derived nutrients, but for most manufacturers, it is simply not cost-effective to make supplements entirely from natural sources. That's why most vitamin and mineral supplements are synthetic, meaning that they are an isolated form of a single nutrient prepared in a laboratory. This doesn't mean, though, as many studies have proved, that they are not well-absorbed by the body. When a vitamin's form does have an impact on its healthfulness, I may specify a natural form.

Example: A natural form of vitamin E, d-alpha-tocopherol, has been shown to have greater bioavailability than the synthetic form, dl-alpha-tocopherol. It is true that some nutrients are better absorbed from food sources than from synthetic sources—so your best bet is to eat a variety of whole foods. Then it's okay to supplement as needed with affordable, high-quality synthetic vitamins.

Erectile Dysfunction Supplements

Mark A. Stengler, NMD, naturopathic physician in private practice, Encinitas, California...adjunct associate clinical professor at the National College of Natural Medicine, Portland, Oregon...author of many books, including *The Natural Physician's Healing Therapies* and coauthor of *Prescription for Natural Cures* (both from Bottom Line Books)...and author of the *Bottom Line/Natural Healing* newsletter.

The market for products that treat erectile dysfunction (ED) is flooded with choices.

Many commonly prescribed drugs, such as *sildenafil* (Viagra), help men achieve and maintain erections by enhancing blood circulation to the penis. But these drugs also can cause serious side effects, such as digestive disturbances, headaches and vision loss. Natural ED remedies also help men achieve and maintain erections by boosting circulation. In addition, they enhance libido, genital sensation and orgasm intensity. But not all natural ED supplements do what their makers claim.

BUYER BEWARE

Perhaps the best-known natural ED supplement is Enzyte. Ads for the product feature "Smilin' Bob," a man with a constant grin—the result of taking Enzyte, of course. The company owner was sentenced to prison for bank fraud conspiracy and other crimes. Enzyte is still on the market. There is nothing dangerous about its ingredients, but there are no studies proving that the product works.

REPUTABLE ED SUPPLEMENTS

If you experience ED, see your doctor to determine the cause. ED can result from clogged blood vessels, a sign of heart disease. If you have heart disease, you need to treat this problem first.

Ask your physician to annually test both your total testosterone level and free testosterone level, the amount available in the bloodstream (not bound to protein). A low total or free testosterone level can cause ED, or it can indicate another problem. Note: ED supplements may not be safe for men with prostate cancer.

Mark Stengler, NMD, recommends the following natural supplements. *Try one product or the other. Do not take both at the same time...*

• **112 Degrees.** The ingredients in 112 Degrees have been shown to support long-term sexual health. *Tribulus terrestris,* a fruit extract regarded in China and Tibet as an aphrodisiac, is thought to enhance sexual desire. *Butea superba,* from the roots of a vine that grows in Thailand, improved erectile function and sexual performance in 82% of men with ED who took 250 milligrams (mg) of the herb daily for three months. *Panax ginseng* is known to increase sexual desire and improve erectile function.

Take two tablets of 112 Degrees once daily—or one tablet twice daily—on an empty stomach. If you have hypertension, have your blood pressure closely monitored. 112 Degrees is available only from the manufacturer (800-901-5526, *www.112degrees.com*).

• **TestoPlex.** This blend of green oat extract, nettle extract, sea buckthorn and oat bran fiber is for men with low levels of free testosterone. Ten clinical trials looked at the effect of green oat extract and found that it increased levels of free testosterone in the body. In one of the studies, men experienced improvement in erectile function and frequency as their free testosterone levels increased. Take four capsules for a total of 2,000 mg once a day in the morning with a full glass of water (available only through health-care professionals, 800-647-6100, *www.xymogen.com*).

Natural Ways to Treat Fibromyalgia

Mark A. Stengler, NMD, naturopathic medical doctor in private practice, Encinitas, California...adjunct associate clinical professor at the National College of Natural Medicine, Portland, Oregon...author of many books, including *The Natural Physician's Healing Therapies* and coauthor of *Prescription for Natural Cures* (both from Bottom Line Books)...and author of the *Bottom Line/ Natural Healing* newsletter.

Pain relief is critically important to the eight to 12 million Americans who suffer from fibromyalgia, a condition characterized by joint and muscle pain and multiple spots on the body that are tender when touched. The pain wears down these patients...and they also must cope with insomnia and severe fatigue. Other symptoms include anxiety...depression...morning stiffness...headaches...abdominal pain...bloating...and constipation.

In the past, many in the medical community dismissed this condition as "all in their patients' heads"—and didn't believe that it was a real medical condition. I never agreed with that. Fibromyalgia is as real as the pain and discomfort it causes. In 2007, for the first time, the FDA approved a drug—*pregabalin* (Lyrica)—to specifically treat the condition. Studies show that this drug is not very effective. I believe that treating fibromyalgia with pharmaceutical drugs, such as Lyrica, or with antidepressants, which also are commonly prescribed, is not the best way for patients to get relief. These drugs have many side effects, including dizziness and coordination problems. I find that many fibromyalgia patients regain their health with natural remedies.

FINDING THE CAUSE

Many patients receive a diagnosis of fibromyalgia from their rheumatologists before coming to see me. Those most at risk are women...people who are 40 to 50 years old... and those with an autoimmune disease, such as lupus or rheumatoid arthritis. I always first test my female patients for hormone deficiencies or imbalances. The results often show low levels of thyroid activity...low progesterone... and not enough of the stress hormone cortisol. With men, I typically first look at thyroid and cortisol levels. Often, once the patient's underlying condition is treated, symptoms disappear completely or are greatly reduced.

NATURAL HELP

Several natural substances can relieve the symptoms of fibromyalgia and reverse the disease's progression. I have used supplements to treat several hundred patients with fibromyalgia. Most of them show signs of improvement within two to four weeks of treatment. After several months, they feel much better. Once they improve, some reduce their doses or no longer need supplements at all. My fibromyalgia patients take most (if not all) of the remedies recommended below. *These supplements help in the following ways...*

BOOST ENERGY

• **D-ribose.** This naturally occurring sugar found in all cells is essential for cellular energy production. Side effects are rare. Although it is a type of sugar, it is safe for people with type 2 diabetes.

Dose: Take 5 grams twice daily in powder form (mixed with water or juice). If taking d-ribose makes you feel light-headed, take it with meals.

• **Coenzyme Q10 (CoQ10).** The antioxidant can increase energy production in cells. CoQ10 is a mild blood thinner, so if you are on blood-thinning medication, consult your physician before taking it.

Dose: Take 200 milligrams (mg) to 300 mg daily with meals.

• **Acetyl-L-carnitine (ALC).** This nutrient can increase cellular energy production.

Dose: Take 500 mg daily on an empty stomach. Cut back on the dosage if it causes digestive upset.

BALANCE NEUROTRANSMITTERS

• **5-hydroxytryptophan (5-HTP).** This form of the amino acid L-tryptophan helps to produce serotonin.

Caution: 5-HTP should not be taken with any psychiatric medications, nor should it be taken by women who are pregnant or breast-feeding. Side effects are rare.

Dose: Take 100 mg three times daily—30 minutes or more apart from eating any food.

• **S-adenosylmethionine (SAMe).**

Caution: SAMe should not be taken if you are on any psychiatric medications. Take either 5-HTP or SAMe. 5-HTP is less expensive, so try it first.

Dose: Take 400 mg twice daily on an empty stomach.

IMPROVE SLEEP

• **Melatonin.** This naturally occurring hormone, derived from serotonin, helps ensure a good night's sleep, which is critical for fibromyalgia patients.

Dose: Start by taking 1 mg 30 minutes before bedtime. If that amount doesn't help you sleep, gradually increase to 3 mg.

RELAX MUSCLES

• **Magnesium.** Take 400 mg to 500 mg daily in two divided doses, with or without food. You can get this total amount from all of your supplement sources added together, including a multivitamin.

• **Vitamin D.** Studies show that people with low levels of vitamin D are at greater risk for fibromyalgia. Taking vitamin D can help relax tight muscles. Your doctor can administer a blood test to check your vitamin D level and to determine the exact dose you need. Most people take 1,000 international units (IU) to 2,000 IU daily.

EATING TO REDUCE PAIN

I recommend that fibromyalgia patients eat an anti-inflammatory diet because this type of diet also will reduce pain. It includes plenty of cold-water fish, such as salmon and sardines... lots of green, leafy and brightly colored vegetables...fruits (berries and apples) and generous amounts of spices with anti-inflammatory properties, such as turmeric, garlic, onions and ginger.

GET MOVING

Exercise can help fibromyalgia patients fight fatigue and pain. In early treatment stages, most people are physically unable to do much exercise because they are in a lot of pain. After that, I advise patients to start walking or using a stationary bike for 10 minutes daily.

REDUCE STRESS

If patients don't exercise, I urge them to find other ways to relax. Stress management is important for all my fibromyalgia patients. Some turn to meditation...prayer...or listening to soft music.

Be Pain Free...Without Drugs

Jill Stansbury, ND, assistant professor and chair of the department of botanical medicine at the National College of Natural Medicine in Portland, Oregon, and medical director of Battle Ground Healing Arts, a naturopathic medical clinic in Battle Ground, Washington. She is the coauthor of *Herbs for Health & Healing.* (Consumer Guide). *http://jillstansbury.net.*

With muscle and joint pain, the cure can often be even worse than the condition.

Reason: Common pain relievers called nonsteroidal anti-inflammatory drugs (NSAIDs)—such as over-the-counter *ibuprofen* (Motrin), *naproxen* (Aleve) and aspirin, as well as prescription *oxaprozin* (Daypro) and controversial *celecoxib* (Celebrex)—have many potentially serious side effects. NSAIDs may...

- **Cause nausea, vomiting, heartburn and gastrointestinal ulcers.**
- **Compromise immunity** by interfering with the body's natural anti-inflammatory chemicals.
- **Thin the blood,** increasing the risk for excessive bleeding.
- **Raise blood pressure.**
- **Lead to kidney or liver failure.**

Much safer: Natural nutritional supplements and topical treatments can reduce chronic or acute pain in muscles and joints. The remedies below are available without a prescription at health-food stores and/or on-line. (As a general precaution, do not use while pregnant or breast-feeding.) The suggested brands are examples from among many good options.

CHRONIC PAIN: SUPPLEMENTS

Nutritional supplements won't provide a quick fix—but when taken daily, they may help relieve persistent pain caused by osteoarthritis (gradual erosion of the cartilage that cushions joints), rheumatoid arthritis (an autoimmune disorder that causes chronic joint inflammation) or an old injury.

You can use any one, two, three or more of the following supplements. Often several are sold together in a combination formula. You may need to use trial-and-error to determine which are most effective for you.

Best: Before starting supplement therapy, it is wise to consult a naturopathic or holistic doctor for usage and dosage guidelines based on your individual sensitivities and symptoms.

If pain is mild, start with the low end of the suggested dosage ranges below to see if you get sufficient relief. For more severe symptoms, start low and work up to the higher end of the ranges if necessary. Dosages may vary by manufacturer, so follow instructions on labels.

Some supplements may cause mild stomach upset and/or gassiness. To minimize this, take with meals and/or cut back the dosage.

Important: Consult your doctor before using supplements if you have any medical problems, such as diabetes or digestive disorders...or if you are taking an antibiotic, blood thinner or medication to control blood sugar or pressure.

Supplements to try...

- **Boswellia,** a resinous plant related to frankincense, blocks production of chemicals that cause pain and swelling.

Recommended brand: Nature's Way Boswellia (800-962-8873, *www.naturesway.com*).

Dosage: One 300 milligram (mg) tablet three times daily.

- **Bromelain** comes from pineapples and has enzymes that can improve circulation and reduce inflammation.

Recommended brand: Thorne Research M.F. Bromelain (800-228-1966, *www.thorne.com*).

- **Glucosamine sulfate** is derived mainly from crustacean shells. Molecularly, it is similar to a natural compound in the human body called *glycosamine glycans,* which is a building block for bones, ligaments and tendons.

Recommended brand: Tyler's Glucosamine Sulfate (800-931-1709, *www.integrativeinc.com*).

Dosage: One 500 mg capsule three times daily.

• **Harpagophytum (devil's claw),** from the sesame family, is an anti-inflammatory and a pain reliever.

Recommended brand: Nature's Way Devil's Claw (800-962-8873, *www.naturesway.com*).

Dosage: One capsule twice daily.

• **Turmeric (curcuma),** the main spice used in curry, limits activity of inflammatory enzymes. Do not supplement with turmeric if you have an ulcer or a problem with your gallbladder or bile duct—it can exacerbate these conditions.

Recommended brand: Gaia Herbs Turmeric Supreme (800-831-7780, *www.gaiaherbs.com*).

Dosage: One capsule once or twice daily.

• **Vitamin D,** which the body synthesizes from sunlight, also is found in fish, eggs and fortified milk. Correcting a deficiency can alleviate musculoskeletal pain. Good brands are available at drugstores and health-food stores.

Dosage: 1,000 international units (IU) to 2,000 IU per day of vitamin D-3 (*cholecalciferol*), the most active form.

ACUTE PAIN: TOPICALS

Oils, ointments and soaks provide quick relief from the pain of muscle strains and arthritis flare-ups. For mild discomfort, try any one of the remedies below...for severe pain, use two or more. Do not use on broken skin or take internally. If skin irritation develops, discontinue use.

• **Arnica,** from a daisylike plant, improves blood flow and reduces inflammation.

To use: For stiff, aching pain, rub a palmful onto the sore area two to three times daily.

Recommended brand: Gaia Herbs Arnica Oil (800-831-7780, *www.gaiaherbs.com*).

• **Castor oil** comes from the castor bean plant. Used topically, it helps blood cells function properly...combats autoimmune diseases...and relieves pain and inflammation.

To use: Just rub a palmful onto skin of the affected area (it can be messy, so you might want to do it at bedtime).

Recommended brand: Frontier Natural Products Co-op Castor Oil (800-669-3275, *www.frontiercoop.com*).

• **Epsom salts** contain magnesium sulfate, which fights infection and inflammation and relaxes muscles.

To use: Fill a basin or bathtub with comfortably hot water, and mix in the desired amount of Epsom salts. The stronger you make the mixture, the more effective it is—try two to three cups of salts per tub of water. Soak the affected area for 15 to 20 minutes once or twice daily, then rinse if desired.

Recommended brand: TheraSoak from Saltworks (800-353-7258, *www.saltworks.us*).

• **Heat rub.** Topical pain relievers (Bengay, Icy Hot) contain organic compounds, such as camphor, menthol and/or *methyl salicylate.* They work by creating a feeling of heat that overrides the nerves' transmission of pain.

To use: Products are available as ointments, creams or skin patches. Follow the manufacturer's instructions for the best amount and frequency of use.

Warning: Methyl salicylate is toxic if used in excess. Do not exceed recommended dosages. Never use multiple heat rubs at once. Do not use with a heating pad or while taking medication from the salicylate family, such as aspirin or antacids.

Recommended brand: Tiger Balm Red (*www.tigerbalm.com*), available at select drugstores and health-food stores.

Are Your Supplements Working or Worthless?

Tod Cooperman, MD, president of ConsumerLab.com, a company that conducts independent testing of health, wellness and nutrition products. General test results are available at no charge to the public. *www.consumerlab.com.* He is also founder of PharmacyChecker.com (*www.pharmacy checker.com*), an evaluator of Internet pharmacies, and editor of *Health, Harm, or Rip-Off? What's Really in Your Vitamins & Supplements* (Bottom Line Books).

Supplement manufacturers will soon be required to test their products for safety and purity. But the US Food and Drug Administration (FDA) has not set a standard for testing...so there's no guarantee that safe and consistent products will soon become available.

Problem: About one out of four supplements contains either less—or more—than the amount of active ingredient listed on the label ...is contaminated with pesticides or heavy metals, such as lead or arsenic...or doesn't disintegrate as it should for proper absorption. Some manufacturers correct such problems when they become aware of them, but others do not.

To learn which supplements were deemed most reliable in testing, we spoke with Tod Cooperman, MD, president of ConsumerLab.com, an independent evaluator of nutritional supplements.*

MULTIVITAMIN/MULTIMINERAL

Supplement makers can legally exceed the tolerable upper intake levels (ULs) for vitamins and minerals—without warning consumers. The UL, set by the National Academies of Science, is the maximum daily intake of a nutrient that is likely to pose no risk for adverse effects in healthy people. Of 32 multivitamin/multiminerals recently tested by ConsumerLab.com, 12 contained at least one nutrient exceeding the UL.

Test results: WEIL Andrew Weil, M.D. Daily Multivitamin...NOW Adam Superior Men's Multi...and Vitamin World Time Release Mega Vita-Min exceeded the UL (35 milligrams [mg] per day) for the B vitamin niacin. One (Swanson Daily Multi-Vitamin & Mineral) contained 100 mg. These niacin amounts were listed on the product labels. Excess niacin can cause skin flushing and tingling...very high amounts can cause liver damage. (Although 1,000 mg of niacin daily can lower cholesterol, such high-dose therapy should be taken only under a doctor's supervision.)

Reliable products include...

- **Kirkland Signature Daily Multi, with Lycopene & Lutein and Calcium.**
- **Centrum Silver Specially Formulated Multivitamin/Multimineral for Adults 50+.**
- **Nutrilite Daily Multivitamin/Multimineral tablets.**

GLUCOSAMINE AND CHONDROITIN

Glucosamine combined with *chondroitin sulfate* slows the joint deterioration and pain associated with osteoarthritis. Glucosamine helps build and repair cartilage, while chondroitin helps preserve the elasticity of cartilage. In a well-publicized study of 1,583 people with knee osteoarthritis, a combination of the supplements helped people with moderate to severe knee pain more effectively than the prescription anti-inflammatory drug *celecoxib* (Celebrex) or a placebo.

Some glucosamine/chondroitin combination supplements skimp on the chondroitin content, probably because it's expensive to produce (chondroitin is predominantly derived from cow cartilage). Of the 20 combination products tested, six contained less chondroitin than listed on the label. Swanson Health Products Premium Brand, while claiming to contain 250 mg of chondroitin sulfate, contained only 20 mg.

Helpful: Products that list an exact amount of "chondroitin sulfate" per dose typically are more reliable than those labeled chondroitin "complex" or "blend." In general, 1,200 mg of chondroitin sulfate and 1,500 mg of glucosamine sulfate or glucosamine hydrochloride daily are recommended for joint pain.

Reliable products include...

- **Puritan's Pride Triple Strength Glucosamine 750 and Chondroitin 600 Dietary Supplement.**
- **Cosamin DS Chondroitin Sulfate Glucosamine HCI 500 mg/Chondroitin Sulfate 400 mg.**
- **Vitamin World Triple Strength Glucosamine 750 mg/Chondroitin 600 mg.**

GINKGO BILOBA

In clinical trials, ginkgo biloba has been shown to fight the cognitive decline associated with dementia as well as circulation problems, ringing in the ears (tinnitus), depression and

*The products listed here have been evaluated by ConsumerLab.com. Other evaluators of supplements include the US Pharmacopeia (USP) and NSF International. Talk to your doctor before taking any nutritional supplement.

asthma. These benefits have been traced to powerful antioxidants that appear to bolster brain activity as well as dilate blood vessels.

Not all ginkgo supplements contain sufficient amounts of these antioxidants.

Of the 13 ginkgo products tested, seven failed because of inadequate amounts of active ingredients. Three of these seven also contained high levels of lead.** All of the lead-contaminated ginkgo supplements contained ginkgo leaf powder and ginkgo leaf extract.

Helpful: To avoid possible lead contamination from ginkgo leaf powder, stick with ginkgo products made only with ginkgo leaf extract. The extraction process appears to remove lead.

The typical daily dosage is 120 mg of the extract, taken in doses of 40 mg or 60 mg over the course of the day. Choose a supplement standardized to contain 24% *flavonol glycosides* and 6% *terpene lactones*—the concentrations used in most clinical trials.

Reliable products include…

- **Nature's Bounty Ginkgo Biloba (120 mg).**
- **Vitamin World Ginkgo Biloba (120 mg).**
- **Puritan's Pride Ginkgo Biloba (60 mg).**

GREEN TEA

Studies show that antioxidants found in green tea—including *epigallocatechin gallate* (EGCG)—may help with the prevention of several cancers, including stomach, lung, liver, breast and colon cancer.

Most green teas are caffeinated, so people who are caffeine sensitive should use the tea with caution.

The seven green tea supplements we tested contained varying amounts of caffeine—from 3 mg per four-capsule dose in one product to 108 mg per four-capsule dose in another. Steeped green tea contains an average of 30 mg of caffeine per eight-ounce cup. (A cup of coffee contains about 100 mg of caffeine.)

**More than 0.5 micrograms per day, as determined by the state of California, the only state to require a label warning for lead contamination in supplements.

Two of the green tea supplements we tested contained extremely high lead levels—Futurebiotics Premium Standardized Green Tea Extract with 4.5 mcg of lead per two-capsule daily dose…and Herbal Select Standardized Green Tea Extract with 6.6 mcg of lead per two-capsule daily dose. A third failed because it didn't provide the EGCG amounts listed on its label.

Caution: Recent reports have linked green tea extracts to liver damage. *Some reliable products include…*

- **Life Extension Mega Green Tea Extract (725 mg per capsule),** 2 mg of caffeine (one capsule).
- **Nature's Bounty Green Tea Extract (315 mg per capsule),** 108 mg of caffeine (four capsules).
- **Pharmanex Tegreen 97 (250 mg per capsule),** 0.75 to 3 mg of caffeine (one to four capsules).

Helpful: Given the high lead content and risks for liver damage, it may be safer to drink green tea. However, the cancer-fighting potency of decaffeinated green tea has not been tested in large-scale studies.

Smart Vitamin Buying

Simeon Margolis, MD, PhD, medical editor, *The Johns Hopkins Medical Letter: Health After 50*, University Health Publishing, 304 Park Ave. S., New York City 10010. *www.johnshopkinshealthalerts.com/health_after_50/.*

To get the most health benefit at the lowest cost from the multivitamin supplements you are taking…

- **Avoid buying "mega-dose" supplements.** They provide far more than 100% of the recommended daily allowance (RDA) for vitamins, anti-oxidants and minerals. Such doses provide no benefit and might prove harmful.
- **Buy a basic multisupplement.** It should provide 100% of the RDA for a large number of vitamins and minerals—a "seniors' formula"

containing an extra amount of vitamin B-12 and lesser amount of iron is fine.

• **Shop by price.** Generic and store brands are just as good as higher-priced name brands, and tablets are as good as capsules.

• **Look for "USP" on the label.** This indicates that the product meets United States Pharmacopeia quality standards.

• **Avoid vitamin combinations that contain herbs, enzymes and hormones.** The benefit of these is unproven and they could be harmful.

• **Don't pay more for unneeded features.** Example one product labeled all natural...timed release...stress formula...starch free...chelated (to promote absorption). They add no value.

Where to Store Your Supplements

Vitamins and supplements lose potency when stored in kitchens and bathrooms.

Reason: Humidity in these rooms can cause slight chemical changes in vitamins and dietary supplements, making them less effective.

Self-defense: Store bottles away from humid areas.

Lisa Mauer, PhD, associate professor of food science, Purdue University, West Lafayette, Indiana, and leader of a study published in *Journal of Agricultural and Food Chemistry.*

SPECIAL REPORT #6

Cooking Secrets That Boost Nutrition

Cooking Secrets That Boost Nutrition

Smarter Cooking

Health-conscious individuals put a lot of time and effort into choosing the most healthful foods.

What too many of us overlook: How various cooking methods affect the nutritional value of these foods. Is it better to boil or steam? Stir-fry or grill? And what about microwaving?

THE VEGGIE FORMULA

You may assume that raw vegetables retain the highest levels of nutrients, but that isn't always true. Cooking—for relatively short durations and at low temperatures—softens the cell walls in many foods, making it easier for the body to remove certain nutrients.

The antioxidant content for most cooked vegetables can be predicted by "time + temperature + water = less nutrition," an equation supported by a recent study published in the *Journal of Food Science.*

In other words, you reduce the amount of antioxidants you get from veggies the longer the cooking time...the higher the cooking temperature...and/or the more water used during the cooking process.

To retain the greatest antioxidant value, the goal is to minimize each of the factors included in the equation when cooking fresh or frozen vegetables. *For example...*

- **Best: griddling.** This is a relatively new-cooking method that is fast becoming favorite of dietitians.

What to do: On a griddle or flat frying pan, spritz a little olive oil (or any other healthful oil), then cook veggies over medium to medium-high heat for about 15 to 20 minutes. This is a long cooking time, but the equation stays low—no water is added, and the vegetables are cooked at a moderate temperature.

Dawn Jackson Blatner, RD, a registered dietitian in private practice in Chicago. A national spokesperson for the American Dietetic Association, she is the author of *The Flexitarian Diet: The Mostly Vegetarian Way to Lose Weight, Be Healthier, Prevent Disease, and Add Years to Your Life* (McGraw-Hill).

If you use a nonstick pan: Add a small spray of olive oil to prevent vegetables from burning. Do not use nonstick pans, such as those coated with Teflon, that have been scratched—they can contaminate your food with toxins.

Smart idea: To avoid *perfluorooctanoic acid* (PFOA), a potentially carcinogenic chemical often used in nonstick pans, consider a ceramic-titanium nonstick pan called Scanpan Green Tek, 877-722-6726, *www.scanpancookware.com*...or Cuisinart Green Gourmet, 800-211-9604, *www.cuisinart.com.*

- **Good: microwaving.** When using a microwave oven, nutritionists recommend adding no more than one tablespoon of water for each cup of vegetables. This helps the equation stay low—the food is typically cooked at a high wattage, but it's for a very short amount of time and very little water is used. Be sure to use a microwave-safe bowl with a cover to retain moisture and help ensure even heating.

Cook on "high" for the shortest amount of time, usually about two to four minutes. Antioxidant levels in carrots, celery and green beans actually improve with microwaving, according to recent research.

- **Good: grilling.** With grilling, the temperature is high, but the cooking time is medium (generally, five to 12 minutes) and no water is used.

Caution: Avoid grilling to the point that veggies become charred—this means that they have been exposed to a high temperature for a long time, possibly depleting vitamins. Grilled vegetables do not contain the carcinogenic *heterocyclic amines* (HCAs) that can be produced when cooking red meat, pork, poultry or fish at high temperatures, such as when grilling or broiling.

- **Good: sautéing or stir-frying.** These methods quickly cook vegetables at medium-to-high temperatures, without water.

Less ideal methods...

- **Steaming.** This method uses a high temperature and cooks vegetables for a medium amount of time in a medium amount of water. Aim to steam only until vegetables are "al dente" (somewhat firm).
- **Baking.** This method generally uses a high temperature and long cooking time, but no water.
- **Slow-cooking.** The temperature is relatively low, but vegetables are cooked for a long time in lots of water. If you like Crock-Pot cooking, make sure you also eat the leftover liquid, which contains much of the leached vitamins.
- **Deep frying.** Despite the fact that water is not typically used and frying time is variable, this high-temperature cooking method is generally considered unhealthy. That's largely because the fat used in cooking penetrates the food, raising its calorie content.
- **Boiling.** This method scores poorly on all three parts of the equation—high temperatures are used, food is cooked for a long time and lots of water is added. In one study, most vegetables tested had their antioxidant value cut by half with boiling.

Better: "Flash-boil" the vegetables for no more than two minutes. Immediately rinse in cold water to stop the cooking process.

BEST WAYS TO COOK MEAT

The minerals and protein in meats are generally stable in heat, so they retain their nutritional value—no matter how you cook them. The most significant concern is to cook meat to a safe internal temperature that will kill pathogens. (Use a meat thermometer to ensure proper cooking temperatures.) *For example...*

Fish: Cook to 145°F or until opaque and flaky—about eight minutes at medium heat for each inch of thickness.

Poultry: Cook to 165°F, until juices run clear.

Beef, pork and lamb: For steaks, roasts and chops, cook to 145°F for medium (center warm and pink)...and to 160°F for well done (brown throughout).

Hamburger: Cook to 160°F to 165°F. One out of every four hamburgers turns brown before it reaches a safe temperature.

Ham: Cook to 160°F if starting from raw... heat to 140°F if starting from precooked.

- **Choose lean cuts of meat and poultry.** If necessary, trim away any fat. If you're grilling, this helps curb the production of carcinogens that can be deposited onto the food by smoke and flare-ups created by dripping fat.

To reduce HCAs: Consider precooking meat or poultry in the microwave, discarding the juice then placing the food onto the grill.

Also helpful: Marinate meat beforehand to reduce potentially cancer-causing HCAs.

Sample marinade: Combine equal parts of oil, white vinegar and water (one-half cup total per pound of meat). Add oregano, basil, garlic, onion, jalapeño pepper, parsley and red pepper. Marinate meats for one hour. Researchers believe that the antioxidants in these herbs help prevent HCAs.

Are You Cooking the Health Out of Your Food?

Richard E. Collins, MD, director of wellness at South Denver Cardiology Associates in Littleton, Colorado. He is board-certified in cardiology and internal medicine, has performed more than 500 cooking demonstrations nationwide and is author of *The Cooking Cardiologist* (Advanced Research) and *Cooking with Heart* (South Denver Cardiology Associates). *www.thecookingcardiologist.com.*

Inflammation is the body's natural, temporary, healing response to infection or injury. But if the process fails to shut down when it should, inflammation becomes chronic—and tissues are injured by excess white blood cells and DNA-damaging free radicals.

Result: Elevated risk for heart disease, cancer, diabetes, osteoporosis, arthritis and other diseases.

Richard E. Collins, MD, "the cooking cardiologist," was recently asked how to prevent chronic inflammation.

His advice: Follow a diet that is rich in immune-strengthening nutrients...and use cooking techniques that neither destroy food's disease-fighting nutrients nor add inflammatory properties to it.

SMART WAYS WITH VEGETABLES

Deeply colored plant foods generally are rich in antioxidants that help combat inflammation by neutralizing free radicals.

Examples: Healthful *flavonoids* are prevalent in deep yellow to purple produce...carotenoids are found in yellow, orange, red and green vegetables.

Exceptions: Despite their light hue, garlic and onions are actually powerful antioxidants.

Unfortunately, these nutrients are easily lost.

For instance: Boiling or poaching vegetables causes nutrients to leach into the cooking water—and get tossed out when that potful of water is discarded. The high heat of frying causes a reaction between carbohydrates and amino acids, creating carcinogenic chemicals called *acrylamides.* And even when healthful food-preparation techniques are used, overcooking destroys nutrients. *Better...*

- **Microwave.** This uses minimal water and preserves flavor (so you won't be tempted to add butter or salt). Slightly moisten vegetables with water, cover and microwave just until crisp-tender.
- **Stir-fry.** In a preheated wok or sauté pan, cook vegetables over medium-high heat for a minute or two in a bit of low-sodium soy sauce.
- **Steam.** This beats boiling, but because steam envelops the food, some nutrients leach out. To "recycle" them, pour that bit of water from the steamer into any soup or sauce.
- **Stew.** Nutrients that leach from the vegetables aren't lost because they stay in the stew sauce.
- **Roast.** Set your oven to 350°F or lower to protect vegetables' nutrients and minimize acrylamides.

BEST METHODS FOR MEAT

When beef, pork, poultry or fish is roasted at 400°F or higher, grilled, broiled or fried, it triggers a chemical reaction that creates inflammatory *heterocyclic amines* (HCAs)—especially when food is exposed to direct flame and/or smoke. At least 17 HCAs are known carcinogens, linked to cancer of the breast, stomach, colon and/or pancreas.

Safest: Roast meat, poultry and fish at 350°F. Avoid overcooking—well-done meats may promote cancer. Also, be sure to avoid undercooking to prevent food poisoning.

If you love to grill: Buy a soapstone grilling stone, one-and-a-quarter inches thick and cut to half the size of your grill. (Stones are sold at kitchen-counter retail stores and also from Dorado Soapstone, 888-500-1905, *www.doradosoapstone.com*). Place it on your grilling rack, then put your food on top of it. Soapstone heats well, doesn't dry out food and gives the flavor of grilling without exposing food to direct flames or smoke.

If you eat bacon: To minimize HCAs, cook bacon in the microwave and take care not to burn it.

THE RIGHT COOKING OILS

Do you cringe when the Food Network chefs sauté in unrefined extra-virgin olive oil? You should. This oil has a very low smoke point (the temperature at which a particular oil turns to smoke) of about 325°F—and when oil smokes, nutrients degrade and free radicals form.

Best: Sauté or stir-fry with refined canola oil, which has a high smoke point. Or use tea seed cooking oil (not tea tree oil)—its smoke point is about 485°F.

Try: Republic of Tea (800-298-4832, *www.republicoftea.com*).

Rule of thumb: If cooking oil starts to smoke, throw it out. Use a laser thermometer (sold at kitchenware stores) to instantly see oil temperature—so you'll know when to turn down the heat.

Best Ways to Cook Your Food

Helen Vlassara, MD, is professor of geriatrics, medicine and molecular medicine, director, division of experimental diabetes and aging, department of geriatric and palliative medicine, Mount Sinai School of Medicine, New York City.

New research from Mount Sinai School of Medicine in New York City suggests it's not only what you eat but how hot you cook it that matters. Subjecting certain foods to prolonged high heat—not only for frying, but also for grilling, roasting, broiling or baking—creates toxic, inflammatory particles. These, in turn, cause the oxidation and inflammation in the body that are associated with such diseases as diabetes, heart disease, kidney disease, Alzheimer's disease and others.

Called *advanced glycation end products* (AGEs), these toxic particles adhere to the arteries, kidneys, brain and joints, where they heighten inflammation. Our typical Western diet, heavy on meat and processed foods and light on plant-based foods, is believed by many scientists to contain at least three times more AGEs than is considered safe.

GOOD NEWS FROM THIS STUDY

It's always exciting when research reveals a way to avoid a common health problem—and this new study does just that. According to the researchers, you can achieve dramatic and quick benefit—within just days—by reducing your intake of AGE-containing foods. Doing this decreases the body's level of inflammation and helps restore its defenses against disease.

The study divided 350-plus participants into three groups—healthy adults between the ages of 18 and 45...an older healthy group, all past age 60...and nine patients with chronic kidney disease (the kidneys are believed to be especially sensitive to AGEs). Participants were randomly assigned to eat either a regular Western diet in which foods were grilled, fried or baked (in other words, loaded with AGEs) or what the researchers called "the AGE-less diet," which included the same foods, only poached, boiled or steamed so that they contained only about half as many AGEs. The two diets were similar in calories and nutrients. After four months, all participants on the AGE-less diet showed a 60% decline in blood levels of AGEs as well as in several other inflammation markers. According to the study's lead author, Helen Vlassara, MD, professor and director of the division of experimental diabetes and aging at Mount Sinai, this indicates that your actual chronological age may not be as significant a factor in aging and health as the AGEs in your food.

A finding that's even more impressive: The patients with kidney disease had a similarly substantial reduction after just one month on the AGE-less diet.

THE HEAT IS ON

How do AGEs get into foods? According to Dr. Vlassara, they develop as a chemical reaction when heat is combined with protein and different sugars, she said—and she noted that meat-rich diets are especially bad, since meats contain high levels of easily oxidizable fat and protein.

There is a third point that is crucial to understand—which is that removing all visible fat when you cook meats doesn't solve the problem. All cells in meats contain not only fat and proteins, but also sugars—some more reactive than others. Therefore, exposure to high heat will still cause AGEs to form in meat at much higher levels than in starch even if you cut away the visible fat. In fact, Dr. Vlassara said that when you see meat brown while cooking, what you're witnessing is the rapid reaction among proteins, fats and those reactive sugars to the heat. And, since they are also animal products, when they are cooked, full-fat milk and cheese also develop high levels of AGEs.

Even worse, manufacturers often add AGE-containing flavor-enhancers or coloring (such as caramel) to processed and packaged foods. A major offender in this category is dark-colored soda. Generally speaking, fast foods and processed/packaged foods also tend to be high in AGEs, which gives us yet another reason to avoid them.

AVOIDING AGES

The good news is, it's not all that difficult to reduce the amount of AGEs in your diet, Dr. Vlassara said. It just requires making some modest changes in the way you prepare food. *Her suggestions...*

MEATS

- **Marinate in an acid-based mixture** (such as vinegar or lemon juice) before cooking, which helps reduce the amount of AGEs produced by heat.

Note: Avoid marinades containing sugar, such as most barbecue and teriyaki sauces.

- **Aim to serve meats rare to medium rare if possible**—for instance, cooking pork to just beyond pink. This is admittedly a balancing act—you want to cook as briefly as possible to minimize development of AGEs, but undercooking carries its own set of dangers.
- **To achieve a brown finish to meats,** Dr. Vlassara suggests cooking on your stovetop with a cover to conserve moisture, and then placing the meat under the broiler for just a few minutes at the end.
- **Use as little fat as possible**—as Dr. Vlassara points out, even healthy olive oil oxidizes at high heat.
- **Water inhibits the formation of AGEs,** so poaching, stewing, steaming or even boiling proteins is best (including fish and eggs).

DAIRY AND OTHER FOODS

- **Avoid bringing dairy products to high temperatures**—for instance, when using milk in sauces or when melting cheese under a broiler. Dr. Vlassara said the less time these foods cook, the better. She added that lower temperatures are preferable, as is increased distance from the heat source.
- **Brief microwaving produces a lower level of AGEs** than broiling, grilling or stovetop cooking, so this is a great way to cook liquids.
- **Plant-based proteins also create dangerous levels of AGEs** when subject to very high heat for long periods—so be aware that there are dangers to even seemingly healthy foods like broiled tofu or roasted nuts.

WHAT ABOUT RESTAURANT FOOD?

Fortunately, the increasingly popular Mediterranean Diet uses lots of foods with low AGEs (including fruits, vegetables, beans and whole grains), so it once again ranks among the healthiest ways that you can eat. This not only provides a good framework for eating at home, it also suggests a wide variety of delicious, healthful, low-AGE dishes that you can order in restaurants. But Dr. Vlassara noted that cooking even these foods at high heat with low hydration is problematic. There's no way around it—cooking at high temperatures is not so hot for your health.

Unsavory Truth About Vegetable Oils

Maggie Ward, MS, RD, LDL, nutrition director of Dr. Mark Hyman's UltraWellness Center, Lenox, Massachusetts. *www.UltraWellnessCenter.com.*

In a recent profile of Whole Foods cofounder and CEO John Mackey, he said that he had given up sugar, most processed foods and vegetable oils. Vegetable oils? Most people think these are healthy, but they're not…here's why.

It used to be that heavy weights were used to squeeze the oil from plants (which is what's really meant by the term "vegetable oil"), but now most manufacturers use heat and chemical solvents, in particular petroleum-derived *hexane*. Both methods end up removing potential health benefits, according to Maggie Ward, MS, RD, LDN, nutrition director of Dr. Mark Hyman's UltraWellness Center in Lenox, Massachusetts. The principle demon is heat. At certain temperatures, heat oxidizes and neutralizes many of the plant's nutrients. This makes the oil rancid (even though you may not be able to tell) and as a result, the oil's healthy antioxidants and essential fatty acids are replaced by destructive free radicals.

Adding insult to injury, most vegetable oils are then refined after extraction—using yet more chemicals and high heat to bleach and deodorize them. This removes color to make the oil look more appealing and erases any rancid smell and taste. The result is oil that is bland enough to add moisture and texture without changing the taste of baked foods, for instance. And the supposed benefit is that cooks can use these oils for frying, because they can be taken to high temperatures without smoking. But the real result of all this processing means that we end up using nutritionally void oil to cook in a way that is inherently unhealthful. And yes, this includes oils such as soybean and canola oil that are marketed as "healthy" and "good for you."

DOES HEALTHFUL OIL EXIST?

Don't throw up your hands in frustration—there are oils that are good for you, produced in ways that preserve their health-giving properties, says Ward. *Here's a list, along with what you need to know about them…*

- **Olive oil.** Olive oil is the leader of the pack when it comes to health, but it requires careful handling. Purchase only olive oil that is cold-pressed (it will say this on the label) and preferably extra-virgin, which will have the most nutrients. When cooking with olive oil, Ward cautions against using heat higher than medium, and if the oil does start to smoke, she says, it should be thrown out. Not only will the heat make it rancid, it will destroy nutrients and create carcinogens, Ward says.

To cook healthfully with olive oil, preheat the pan for up to a minute and then add the food and oil at the same time rather than starting with the oil alone. This prevents overheating and provides a bonus—the food better absorbs the oil's healthy essential fatty acids. For added flavor and health, sprinkle a bit of olive oil over the food when you have finished cooking.

To store olive oil: Keep it in a dark glass bottle or any opaque container in your cabinet or on the counter—no need to refrigerate unless your kitchen is exceptionally warm.

- **Tropical oils.** Coconut and, to a lesser degree, palm oil have had a health resurgence in recent years. As saturated fats, these used to be considered unhealthy for the heart, but this type of oil is now recognized by physicians and scientists as necessary and good for you (though not in excess). These oils will not oxidize, so you can cook with them at higher temperatures.

Storage for coconut and palm oils: Since these oils are not sensitive to temperature or light, it is fine to store them on the counter or in the pantry.

- **Seed and nut oils.** Some seed and nut oils have become popular as seasoning added to salads and other dishes after cooking. Sesame oil, for example, has plenty of antioxidants, and Ward says that unrefined sesame oil retains more of its nutrients because the seeds are easy to press. However, seed and nut oils turn rancid quickly (even when kept cool), so it is best to buy small quantities that you can use within a few weeks. Sniff the oil before using—toss it if it no longer smells fresh.

Nut and seed oil storage: Refrigerate in dark bottles.

Salt-Free Seasoning Made Easy

Judith Wylie-Rosett, EdD, RD, head for health behavior and nutrition research in the department of epidemiology and population health at Albert Einstein College of Medicine in New York City. She is the author of *The Complete Weight Loss Workbook: Proven Techniques for Controlling Weight-Related Health Problems* (American Diabetes Association) and has published more than 130 journal articles on nutrition and health.

Have you had much luck in getting your loved ones (not to mention yourself) to put down the saltshaker? Many are more bothered by the taste of bland, boring food than by the increased threat of a heart attack or stroke.

They are not alone, of course. More than half of Americans age 60 and older have hypertension. If you or someone you cook for is among them, you may have tried to fool the taste buds with a commercial salt substitute but found the flavor too bitter.

Well, take heart. Nutrition researcher Judith Wylie-Rosett, EdD, RD, whose book *The Complete Weight Loss Workbook* includes many health-promoting recipes, suggested some much better ways to put zing into low-salt foods. *To get started...*

- **It can take a lot of seasoning to make up for the missing salt**—so when you drop salt from a recipe, try doubling one or more of the other seasonings the recipe calls for.
- **For maximum flavor from herbs and spices, opt for fresh rather than dried.**
- **Choose herb-infused oils and vinegars instead of unflavored ones.**

TASTY, SALT-FREE WAYS TO SPICE UP

- **Beef.** For seasoning that stands up to red meat's strong flavor, marinate beef for two to three hours in pineapple juice or orange juice mixed with balsamic vinegar, red wine, diced onions and/or chopped garlic.
- **Chicken.** For delicate-flavored lemon chicken, add chopped tarragon, which is subtly bittersweet and minty. Robust chicken parmigiana needs more aggressive seasonings, such as fennel, basil, rosemary, garlic and/or oregano. For stews, add a bay leaf (remove before eating) plus mustard, marjoram and freshly ground black pepper...or use strong spices, such as cumin, turmeric and/or ginger.
- **Fish.** Complement mild-flavored white fish with the tangy taste of yogurt. Mix plain lowfat or nonfat yogurt with dill, ginger, mustard and garlic, then add one tablespoon of mayonnaise per cup of yogurt to keep the yogurt from separating. Use this as a marinade... or serve with the fish as a sauce. Fatty fish (mackerel, bluefish) have a strong flavor that blends well with the hearty taste of curry, lemon pepper and garlic.
- **Pasta.** Instead of salting the cooking water, keep pasta from sticking by using extra cooking water and a splash of flavored olive oil. Drain pasta one minute earlier than you normally would, return it to the pot, stir in whatever sauce you're going to use and cook them together for that final minute—so the pasta absorbs more flavor from the sauce.
- **Soups.** For delicate-flavored soups, such as chicken soup, use chopped sage, parsley and thyme to enhance but not overwhelm the flavor. To give zest to hearty-tasting soups, add a splash of balsamic vinegar and/or wine when the soup is almost done.
- **Vegetables.** Stir together two or more types of cooked veggies before serving—they taste more interesting that way than alone—and boost flavor with a generous amount of fresh-squeezed lemon juice. Simmer root vegetables in reduced-fat coconut milk mixed with curry. Dress salads with herb-infused olive or sunflower oil...champagne vinegar or vinegar made from sweeter fruits (pears, figs, raspberries)...and some fresh flat-leaf parsley, chervil or tarragon.

Salt? Who needs it?

Raw vs. Cooked Spinach

Eat a wide variety of vegetables, prepared in various ways, including raw and cooked spinach. Cooking vegetables such as spinach can provide higher levels of antioxidants, such as carotenoids. Cook in a flat skillet to retain the highest amounts of antioxidants. Other nutrients don't fare as well during cooking. To retain the most vitamin C in vegetables high in the vitamin, such as broccoli, cook for the shortest time and with little water.

Mark A. Stengler, NMD, naturopathic medical doctor in private practice, Encinitas, California...adjunct associate clinical professor at the National College of Natural Medicine, Portland, Oregon...author of many books, including *The Natural Physician's Healing Therapies* and coauthor of *Prescription for Natural Cures* (both from Bottom Line Books)...and author of the *Bottom Line/ Natural Healing* newsletter.

Good Health...and No Cooking...From a Raw Food Diet

Natalia Rose, CN, author of *The Raw Food Detox Diet* (HarperCollins).

Nowadays it's not considered all that unusual to hear someone declare himself a raw-food devotee and announce he has decided to stop cooking...altogether. The ranks of raw foodists are growing as people search for ways to "greenify" their lives.

IS COOKING BAD FOR YOUR HEALTH?

Health is usually cited as the primary motivator for this lifestyle change based on the core belief that heating any food to a temperature higher than 116°F destroys its natural enzymes, thereby making it impossible for the body to fully absorb the nutrients. Raw foodists say that cooking destroys many nutrients and claim that cooking foods damages the molecular structure as well, rendering foods "toxic." The purported rewards of eating a raw diet are improved energy and health, weight loss, detoxification of the body, better immune system, improved mental status, and more.

Natalia Rose, CN (clinical nutritionist), author of *The Raw Food Detox Diet*, helps people "cleanse their bodies" to improve health and metabolism through a careful eating program that includes many raw foods. (Actually, few raw foodists go completely raw—most eat anywhere from 75% to 90% raw.) Interestingly, she thinks many fanatical raw foodists have vilified cooked vegetables while eating too many non-cleansing raw foods such as nuts, dried foods, coconut oil and other fats that they call "healthful" in place of fruits and vegetables. A popular piece of equipment among raw foodists is a food dehydrator because it mimics the taste, texture and fullness of cooked foods. However, says Rose, foods processed this way are very dense and hard on the digestive system, causing constipation, food fermentation and the breeding of yeast and bacteria. The point is not to set a goal of eating only raw foods, but rather to eat a diet with a high percentage of fruits and vegetables, healthy in part because they contain lots of water that cleanses the cells.

In her view, the goal should be to eat in a way that supports superb digestion and a clean system—not to focus on raw foods as a way of life. In fact, she says, cooked foods are not necessarily harmful or difficult to digest—they can actually help your body cleanse at a more natural pace. It also makes for a lifestyle that is easier socially and emotionally.

BENEFITS OF A RAW DIET

According to Rose, the digestive system is prone to get bogged down by the residue of waste left over from processed and incompletely digested foods that may remain in the large intestine. To have a clean system, she says, you must rid the body of that waste, which is where raw fruits and vegetables come in. Raw produce alkalizes the body, helps remove built-up waste and provides plentiful enzymes necessary for healthy functioning. Building a diet around foods that clear the system appropriately promotes health so you feel "super good," in her words.

Rose's specialty is developing dietary detox programs that will help people feel exactly that—super good. She is adamant that it takes time to transition from a diet of mostly cooked and processed foods to one that is fresh and mostly raw, however. This is why her program has five levels of plans.

Level five has plentiful amounts of raw fruits and vegetables, some cooked animal products and vegetables, but no processed foods or sugar, while level one comes close to 100% raw. But, she reiterates the importance of a gradual transition. Along the way, Rose says, many discover they don't want to go all the way to level one, finding it extreme. Instead they find they are comfortable and feel good eating somewhere in the middle range.

HOW TO FEEL "SUPER GOOD"

If your goals are to lose weight, gain energy and clean out your digestive system, Rose has basic dietary advice that's easy to implement immediately. She characterizes her approach as a transition plan, a convenient way to segue from a mainstream diet to a cleansing one.

Here's how to get going...

- **Food combining is at the core of her program for proper and prompt digestion.** Foods are separated into five categories—fruit, vegetables, animal products (including dairy products from cows, goats and eggs), starch (including whole grains and cooked starchy vegetables such as sweet potatoes and winter squash), and seeds, nuts and dried fruits. Always eat fruits separate from all other foods —do not eat anything else for at least 20 minutes afterward and avoid fruit for two to three hours after eating other foods. Vegetables are neutral and can be eaten along with anything but fruit.
- **Eat light to heavy**—start the day with light food such as fresh fruits and eat the heaviest foods during dinner, which could be salad, steamed fish and vegetables. Though this advice runs counter to what we've always heard, Rose says it is because the body is in elimination mode in the morning—eating heavy foods then forces the body to digest instead of eliminate.
- **For the same reason, breakfast should be fresh vegetable juice or fresh whole fruit.** (For juicing, Rose likes the Breville juicers, *www.brevilleusa.com.*)
- **Lunch generally consists of an assortment of vegetables and lean protein.** Rose suggests a hearty raw vegetable salad as the focal point of lunch—it can be topped with grilled chicken, tuna or salmon. You can also pair the salad with a starch such as sweet potato or avocado or with a sandwich on high-quality sprouted grain bread. An omelet is another option.
- **Dinner combines another raw vegetable salad (including goat cheese if you wish), and often something cooked**—for instance, steamed vegetables and fish, an omelet, or whole-grain pasta with vegetables or organic marinara sauce.

Minimize snacking and try to stick mostly to raw vegetables (the quantities are unlimited). For a treat, you can enjoy several one-inch squares of dark chocolate a day (Green & Black's Organic or others that are at least 70% cocoa) and one glass of wine—either red or white.

Gourmet Cooking Secrets for People with Diabetes

Chris Smith, the Diabetic Chef, an executive chef working in the healthcare field. He was diagnosed with type 1 diabetes at age 24. Author of two cookbooks, *Cooking With the Diabetic Chef* and *The Diabetic Chef's Year-Round Cookbook* (both from American Diabetes Association), he lectures widely about cooking for people with diabetes.

Can people with diabetes eat healthfully and enjoy their meals at the same time? The answer is a resounding "yes," says Chris Smith, author of *The Diabetic Chef's Year-Round Cookbook* (American Diabetes Association). Smith uses fresh, seasonal ingredients to create healthy, interesting meals full of flavor for individuals with diabetes and everyone else at the table, while reducing the salt, sugar and fat that many have come to rely upon to add taste.

HEALTHY EATING...WITH DIABETES

Just like the rest of us, people with diabetes should eat nutritious meals that are low in fat (especially saturated and trans fat), moderate in salt and very sparing in sugar, while emphasizing whole grains, vegetables and fruit. However, because people with diabetes are at a greater risk for life-threatening complications such as hypertension, heart disease and stroke, it's particularly important that they keep blood glucose control while maintaining normal levels of blood pressure and blood lipids (cholesterol). It can be challenging to do all that while still preparing flavorful and appealing food. Here the Diabetic Chef shares his secrets for preparing foods that are appropriate for people with diabetes and delicious enough for everyone.

HERBS AND SPICES ARE ESSENTIAL

Liven up your meals with garden-fresh herbs, many of which are available year-round. Fresh herbs are densely packed with flavor. You can use herbs in a variety of ways throughout the seasons.

• **Fine herbs, such as thyme, oregano, dill, basil and chives,** are usually available in the spring and summer. These should be added as a finish (at the end of the cooking process) to release their delicate flavors and aromatic qualities. "Use fresh basil with summer tomatoes and olive oil for pasta, or as a finish to a tomato sauce," said Smith. "Use chives as a delicate finish to soups, salads and sauces."

• **Hearty herbs (rosemary, sage),** available year-round, can be added earlier on in the cooking process. Use them with stews, soups and Crock-Pot dishes. They can withstand the heat of cooking without losing flavor and, in fact, the longer they're cooked, the more mellow and flavorful they are, says Smith.

• **Dried herbs** must be rehydrated, so use at the beginning of the cooking process (adding as you sauté onions for a sauce, for example). Your homemade tomato sauce with dried oregano and basil tastes better the next day as the flavor of the dried herbs fully blooms and combines with the other ingredients.

Herb typically describes the leaves of a plant, while spices are derived from any other part—including the root, seeds, bark or buds. Spices can be used to create a medley of flavors and can be evocative of different types of ethnic cuisines. "Spices bring great diversity to food," Smith says.

OTHER TIPS FOR HEALTHFUL EATING

Overall, Smith points out that healthful eating is a matter of practicing what he calls "Nutritional MVP," which stands for moderation, variety and portion control.

From his cookbook, another suggestion is to learn how to do template cooking. Template cooking is taking one recipe and adapting it in different ways by using the same cooking method but substituting different ingredients, says Smith. "It gives you the freedom to be creative, which is the essence of good cooking." It also brings much-needed diversity to meals, so you are not forever serving the same old thing. One example of a template recipe is the Simple Chicken Breast (see the next page). "There are only seven ingredients in this recipe but you can vary it with fresh, seasonal ingredients," says Smith. "For instance, in springtime you can exchange the olive oil for sesame oil and use lemon grass rather than garlic to create an Asian flavor. In summer, substitute fresh cilantro for the rosemary."

Try different cooking techniques to bring out the essence of foods.

• **Grill, broil, roast, sauté or steam food to enhance flavor without added fat or salt.** Slow-roast vegetables with a drizzle of olive oil in a 400-degree oven to bring out their true flavors. Many develop a natural sweetness when roasted. Season with garlic or add herbs to vary the taste. Rather than sautéing garlic or onions with butter or oil before adding them to soups or stews, try roasting in the oven.

• **Marinate foods in a few ingredients.** "The herbs, lemon and spice in the Simple Chicken Breast recipe create a vibrant flavor, and the extra-virgin olive oil allows the herbs and spices to reach their full bouquet," said Smith.

• **Sear meat (brown on both sides in a pan for a few minutes before placing it in the oven) to enhance flavor without adding extra fat or salt.** "Any kind and cut of meat can be seared," said Smith.

•**Pair dishes with colorful sides.** Instead of a plate full of brown items such as chicken and rice, liven up your plate with deeply colored fruits and vegetables that add variety and important phytonutrients (components of fruits and vegetables that are thought to promote health) to your diet.

•**Keep the pantry stocked with these healthy ingredients.**

Oils: extra-virgin olive oil, sesame oil, peanut oil and grapeseed oil.

Vinegars: balsamic, champagne, rice and aged sherry vinegar.

Essential spices: cayenne pepper, chili powder, cinnamon, mustard, nutmeg, paprika and pepper.

Essential dry herbs: bay leaves, dill, basil, oregano, rosemary, thyme and sage.

Other essential products: chicken, vegetable and beef broth, dried beans, whole gluten-free grains such as quinoa and amaranth.

Essential fresh ingredients: lemons, limes, oranges, garlic, onions, shallots, carrots, tomatoes, potatoes, mushrooms, butter (salt free), sour cream (fat free), eggs, hard cheeses (Parmesan and Romano), mustard (grain, Dijon), capers and olives.

TEMPLATE RECIPE: SIMPLE CHICKEN BREAST

Serves 4

4 chicken breast halves
1 tablespoon extra-virgin olive oil
1 tablespoon dried rosemary
1 tablespoon poultry seasoning
1 teaspoon salt-free lemon pepper
1 tablespoon minced garlic
½ teaspoon red pepper flakes
Cooking spray

1. In medium bowl, combine all ingredients and place chicken breasts in it. Cover and refrigerate 1 hour.

2. Preheat oven to 375°F.

3. Preheat sauté pan to medium-high heat. Spray pan with cooking spray. Add chicken breast to pan and sear to desired color, about 10 seconds, then turn over and sear other side.

4. When both sides are seared, remove chicken from pan and place in a baking dish or cookie sheet. Do not cover. Place in oven. Cook meat until internal temperature reads 165°F. When chicken is done, remove from oven and let rest for two to four minutes.

For more tips from Chef Smith go to: *www.thediabeticchef.com.*

The Healthy Connoisseur's Guide to Green Tea

Lester A. Mitscher, PhD, professor and former chair of medicinal chemistry, University of Kansas, Lawrence, and coauthor of *The Green Tea Book* (Avery).

The world's most healthful beverage may be green tea. Reason: It is rich in *catechins*, potent antioxidant plant chemicals that neutralize cell-damaging free radicals, fight bacteria and ease inflammation. The most beneficial catechin in green tea is *epigallocatechin gallate* (EGCG).

Studies suggest that green tea protects against heart disease by reducing blood pressure, cholesterol and blood clotting...cancer by blocking tumors' blood supply...diabetes by improving the cells' response to insulin... Alzheimer's disease and Parkinson's disease by reducing brain-damaging proteins...arthritis and osteoporosis by slowing breakdown of cartilage and bone...gastrointestinal disorders by improving liver function...obesity by increasing metabolism...and cavities, gum disease and bad breath by destroying bacteria in the mouth.

All tea (except herbal) comes from the *Camellia sinensis* plant. Variations in taste are due to where the tea is grown and how it is processed (just as with wine). Once picked, tea leaves start to oxidize, darkening like a sliced apple. Then leaves are heated to halt oxidation. Black tea is the most oxidized...oolong less so...green tea only slightly. Because oxidation destroys catechins, black tea typically has less than half the antioxidant power of green tea. (Unoxidized white tea has slightly more antioxidants than green tea, but it costs more and is less readily available.) *To maximize green tea's health benefits and flavor...*

• **Drink three to six eight-ounce cups daily.** Check with your doctor first if you take blood-thinning medication, such as *warfarin* (Coumadin)—tea may alter the drug's effects.

• **The larger the leaf fragments, the higher the antioxidant content**—so choose loose tea with recognizable leaf tips, such as the Sencha variety from Japan. Tea bags are convenient but contain smaller fragments. If you like bottled tea, compare labels and pick one high in EGCG.

• **To avoid possible contamination with lead, pesticides or other toxins, opt for organic teas.**

• **Antioxidants degrade over time, so buy only as much green tea as you can use within six months.** Choose light-colored loose leaves with no moldy scent. With tea bags and bottles, check for a "use by" date on labels. Store tea leaves and bags in an airtight, opaque container along with a desiccant packet ($3.99 at *www.containerstore.com*). Place in a cool, dry place or refrigerate.

• **Brew using water that is not quite boiling.** Steep for no more than three minutes to avoid bitterness, using a covered china, glass or stainless steel pot or cup. Strain loose leaves before drinking to avoid grittiness. Do not reuse leaves or bags—reused tea is more bitter and lower in antioxidants.

• **Citrus juice may increase catechins' absorption** from the digestive tract, so add lemon if you like. Do not add milk—its proteins may decrease catechin absorption. Herbal or fruit flavoring does not affect levels of antioxidants in the tea.

• **If you prefer decaffeinated tea, check labels and choose a brand that uses the catechin-sparing carbon dioxide method of decaffeination, not the ethyl acetate method.**

If you don't care for the taste of green tea, try an extract with a catechin content of 65% or more. Do not exceed the manufacturer's dosage guidelines—a laboratory study suggests that daily megadoses of EGCG may promote tumor growth.